MRCPsych Paper I One-Best-Item MCQs

MRCPsych Paper I
One-Best-Item MCQs
with answers explained

DAVID BROWNE
MB BCh BAO MRCPsych
Postgraduate Certificate in Medical Education Diploma in Management
Consultant Psychiatrist s.i. Rehabilitation
Donegal Mental Health Services

BRENDA WRIGHT
MB BCh BAO MRCPsych MFFLM
Consultant Forensic Psychiatrist
National Forensic Mental Health Service

GUY MOLYNEUX
MB BCH BAO MRCPsych Postgraduate Diploma in CBT
Diploma in Management
Consultant Psychiatrist
Health Service Executive, Dublin

MOHAMED AHMED
MMedSc MBBS MRCPsych DCP
Senior Registrar in General Adult Psychiatry in Clare MHS
Honorary Research Fellow, Department of Psychiatry
National University of Ireland, Galway

IJAZ HUSSAIN
MMedSc MBBS MRCPsych DCP
Senior Registrar in General Adult Psychiatry
North Tipperary Mental Health Services

BANGARU RAJU
MD MBA BS MRCPsych DPM
Consultant Psychiatrist, West Blanchardstown Sector
Clinical Tutor, Dublin Northwest Mental Health Services
Programme Co-ordinator, RCSI Postgraduate Psychiatric Training Programme

MICHAEL REILLY
MB BCh BAO MRCPsych Diploma in Management
Consultant Psychiatrist s.i. Rehabilitation
Sligo Leitrim Mental Health Service

Radcliffe Publishing
Oxford • New York

WM 18
Browne

H0903626

Radcliffe Publishing Ltd
18 Marcham Road
Abingdon
Oxon OX14 1AA
United Kingdom

www.radcliffe-oxford.com
Electronic catalogue and worldwide online ordering facility.

British Library Cataloguing in Publication Data

A catalogue record for this book is available from the British Library.

ISBN-13: 978 184619 008 7

The paper used for the text pages of this book is FSC certified. FSC (The Forest Stewardship Council) is an international network to promote responsible management of the world's forests.

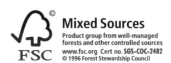

Mixed Sources
Product group from well-managed forests and other controlled sources
www.fsc.org Cert no. SGS-COC-2482
© 1996 Forest Stewardship Council

FSC

Typeset by Pindar NZ, Auckland, New Zealand
Printed and bound by TJI Digital, Padstow, Cornwall, UK

Contents

Preface

Change has come again to the Royal College of Psychiatrists' MRCPsych examinations. The past decade has seen several revisions in the examinations but the latest changes have been the most radical. We have attempted to help trainees keep pace with some of these changes with this new 'one-best-item-from-five' style multiple-choice question book for the new MRCPsych Paper I. The 'old' MRCPsych examination with its individual statement questions (ISQs) is no longer. The examination is now a three-part written examination and Clinical Assessment of Skills and Competencies (CASC). This three-paper format has changed the focus of the 'new' MRCPsych Paper I.

The new MRCPsych Paper I consists of two-thirds 'one-best-item-from-five' style questions and one-third extended matching items (EMIs). For experience with EMIs, the reader is encouraged to consult the related publication *Extended Matching Items for the MRCPsych Part 1*.[1] The curriculum for the new Paper I has a somewhat narrower focus than the old MRCPsych Part I, but there are additional areas to be studied, e.g. basic ethics, philosophy and history of psychiatry, along with stigma and culture.[2]

One difficulty that can arise from using MCQ books is getting too familiar with one or two authors' styles and finding a difference from these and the questions in the real examination. The Royal College of Psychiatrists of course uses many authors to build large banks of questions for the examinations. We have taken the approach in this book of having multiple authors with different writing styles and interests to compose a variety of one-best-item MCQs. We believe this gives a variety of question styles which will approximate more closely the examination paper itself.

We have attempted to vary the level of difficulty of the questions for the same reason, ranging from straightforward to very difficult. Another decision has been to keep the MCQs 'mixed up', so that one does not just do, say, psychology questions alone for 10 pages. This is to ensure candidates are encouraged to continue studying all relevant subjects equally throughout rather than sequentially. Particular focus has been given to areas of the curriculum that are both important and that lend themselves well to one-best-item

MCQs, e.g. defence mechanisms, transcultural psychiatry or diagnostic criteria.

Our aim with this book is to provide 500 questions of the one-best-item style MCQs to help familiarise candidates with this type of MCQ and to help direct their study. The answers to all the questions are provided on the succeeding page, with explanations given for answers as to why a particular answer is the 'best' of the items presented. The answers are referenced to textbooks which deal with the subject matter. Readers can thus check why a given answer is thought to be preferred and further information on the topic can be accessed. In the early stages of Paper I examination preparation, a 'wrong' answer is very useful in prompting areas where further study is required. Closer to the examination date, the book can be used to test yourself under examination conditions.

The reading list recommended by the Royal College of Psychiatrists for MRCPsych examination preparation is a broad and a somewhat daunting list on first inspection. We have tried as much as possible to use a wide range of commonly used texts in writing these questions to aid your preparation for the examination. The most frequently referenced textbooks used are our recommended reading.

It is crucial in answering the questions to realise one-best-item MCQs are related to EMIs in that all items can be correct: you are required to choose the *best* answer from these. Therefore when you see a good answer to the question stem, check again to see if there is a better one.

It just remains for us to wish you success in the MRCPsych Paper I examination and in your career in Psychiatry!

DB
MR
Dublin & Sligo
April 2009

References

1 Reilly M, Raju B. *Extended Matching Items for the MRCPsych Part 1*. Oxford: Radcliffe Publishing; 2004.
2 www.rcpsych.ac.uk/exams/about/mrcpsychpaper1.aspx

About the authors

David Browne began basic specialist training in Psychiatry in 1999 on the Western Health Board Psychiatric Training Scheme. Having completed the MRCPsych in 2002, he carried out research in the area of epidemiology of first-episode and prevalent psychoses. He has an interest in medical education and training, was a member of the Royal College of Psychiatrists, Psychiatric Training Committee from 2003 to 2005, and is well versed in the recent changes to the MRCPsych examination. He completed a Post Graduate Certificate in Medical Education with Queens University, Belfast. In 2002 he co-authored an MCQ book for MRCPsych examination preparation, *MCQs for the New MRCPsych Part II*. He works as a Consultant Psychiatrist with a special interest in Rehabilitation in the northwest of Ireland.

Brenda Wright qualified in medicine from UCD in 1997. She completed her psychiatric training with the St John of God Rotation in Dublin, having obtained her Membership of the Royal College of Psychiatry in 2002. She is currently a Consultant in Forensic Psychiatry with the National Forensic Mental Health Service. She previously held the post of Lecturer in Forensic Psychiatry with the National University of Ireland, Trinity College, Dublin. She is a member of the Faculty of Forensic and Legal Medicine of the Royal College of Physicians. She has done research particularly in the areas of psychiatric morbidity in prison and cognitive patterns in sex offenders.

Guy Molyneux is a consultant General Adult Psychiatrist working in Dublin for the HSE. He graduated from Trinity College, Dublin in 1996 and completed his psychiatric training (General Adult and Old Age Psychiatry) in Ireland. He was the Lecturer in Psychiatry at the Royal College of Surgeons in Ireland in 2004 and enjoyed serving on the college trainee and senior registrar steering committees. His clinical interests include Cognitive Psychotherapy and home-based treatment. His research interests include carer burden: a presentation of his paper on the subject won first prize at the 12th Annual Congress of the International Psychogeriatric Association.

Mohamed Ahmed graduated in 1996 and worked in Jordan, Sudan and Saudi Arabia prior to completing his basic psychiatric training on the Western Health Board Psychiatric Training Scheme. He then completed a higher diploma in clinical teaching and has been actively participating in teaching postgraduate psychiatric trainees in the west of Ireland. His special interests are transcultural psychiatry, neuroimaging and metabolic disorders in schizophrenia.

Ijaz Hussain graduated in 1999 and worked in Ireland. He completed his basic psychiatric training on the Western Health Board Psychiatric Training Scheme. He is currently a Senior Registrar in general adult psychiatry and Honorary Lecturer with the National University of Ireland, Galway. He developed an interest in teaching as an SHO and worked as a Clinical Lecturer with the Department of Psychiatry, National University of Ireland, Galway. He has successfully organised courses for the MRCPsych exam under the old and new curriculum, and is experienced in the recent changes in psychiatric training.

Bangaru Raju qualified in medicine from the University of Madras, India in 1981. Between 1981 and 1986 he completed basic psychiatric training and higher psychiatric training at the Institute of Psychiatry in Madras. He worked as Assistant Professor of Psychiatry in the University of Madras for nine years. Subsequently he completed basic specialist training in Psychiatry in 1999 on the Western Health Board Psychiatric Training Scheme. His MD (Madras) thesis was on the dexamethasone suppression test. He then worked as Temporary Consultant of Psychiatry of Old Age for two years. He completed higher psychiatric training in the Limerick Mental Health Services, Dublin Northwest Mental Health Services and in the National Forensic Psychiatric Services, Ireland. He has completed an MBA in Health Service Management on the UCD/RCSI programme. He has co-authored a number of MCQ books for the MRCPsych examinations: *MCQs for the New MRCPsych Part I, MCQs for the New MRCPsych Part II* and *Extended Matching Items for the MRCPsych Part 1.* His interests include medical education, forensic psychiatry, mood disorders and administration. Since 2005 he has worked as a Consultant Psychiatrist with the Dublin Northwest Area Psychiatric Services. Since 2006 he has been the Clinical Tutor in Psychiatry of Dublin Northwest Area and since 2007 he has been the Programme Co-ordinator of RCSI Postgraduate Psychiatric Training Programme. He is the current chair of Continuing Professional Development sub-committee of The Irish College of Psychiatrists.

Michael Reilly qualified in medicine from UCD in 1995. He completed basic specialist training in Psychiatry in 1999 on the Western Health Board Psychiatric Training Scheme. He spent two years researching biological and clinical correlates of suicidal behaviour as part of the INSURE Collaborative

Project on suicidal behaviour. He completed higher psychiatric training in the Cavan/Monaghan Mental Health Services and in the Department of Psychiatry, University College Hospital, Galway. He has co-authored a number of MCQ books for the MRCPsych examinations: *MCQs for the New MRCPsych Part I, MCQs for the New MRCPsych Part II* and *Extended Matching Items for the MRCPsych Part 1*. His interests include medical education, psychiatric ethics and the psycho-social treatment of severe and enduring mental illness. Since 2005 he has worked as a Consultant Psychiatrist with a special interest in Rehabilitation in the northwest of Ireland.

Acknowledgements

We wish to express our gratitude to various groups who have helped us in some shape or form to produce this book:

- Ms Mary Goodwin for her unstinting advice on word processing, orthography and layout. The book looks so much better thanks to your input!
- Dr Udeme E Akpan for his contribution with the following MCQs: 204, 208, 214, 218, 224, 228, 234, 238, 244, 248, 254, 258, 264, 268, 274, 278, 284, 288, 294, 298. Udeme is a graduate of Obafemi Awolowo University, Ile-Ife, Nigeria. He is currently a registrar with the Sligo/Leitrim Mental Health Service. His main area of academic interest is in affective neurosciences. He is a travel enthusiast and a lover of life.
- Our colleagues and teachers over the years for their support.
- Some other people we would like to acknowledge individually:
  - **DB:** Jane and Emily, the Browne and Daly families.
  - **GM:** I'd like to thank my wife Gill, for unending support and for assistance editing my contribution.
  - **MA:** To my family: Nasrein and Siddig.
  - **BR:** To my wife Prabha and daughters Dhivya and Deepa.
  - **MR:** To the baggage: Samantha, Nicole and Caoimhe, Eileen and Elizabeth and the Fox family.

Questions and Answers

1 A 25-year-old woman with a long history of treatment for schizoaffective disorder presents to the outpatient department. She has been referred by her GP who reports that she is six weeks' pregnant. He is requesting a review of her medication with regard to teratogenicity. Which of the following medications needs to be most urgently reviewed?

A. Carbamazepine.

B. Clonazepam.

C. Fluoxetine.

D. Olanzapine.

E. Sodium valproate.

2 A well-groomed 30-year-old woman presents to an A&E department in a city 150 km distant from her home. She informs the doctor that she has no memory of getting to the city. Physical examination reveals no organic abnormality. Which of the following ICD-10 diagnoses is the most likely in this case?

A. Amnesia.

B. Dissociative amnesia.

C. Dissociative fugue.

D. Dissociative stupor.

E. Trance disorder.

3 A 30-year-old man presents with depressive symptoms. A possible cause could be which of the following?

A. Brucellosis.

B. Cushing's syndrome.

C. Hepatitis.

D. Hypothyroidism.

E. All of the above.

4 A 26-year-old woman with schizophrenia was punched in the abdomen by another patient on the ward. When examined by the duty SHO, she stated: 'The pain in my tummy is the result of an implanted exploding device being controlled by Al Qaeda terrorists in the nurses' station.' The phenomenological term that closest fits her experience is:

A. Delusional perception.

B. Haptic hallucination.

C. Paranoid delusion.

D. Passivity of volition.

E. Somatic passivity.

1 **Answer: E.** Ideally all medication should be avoided in pregnancy. Polypharmacy should particularly be avoided. Both sodium valproate and carbamazepine are to be avoided in pregnancy, and both have a proven causal link with foetal abnormalities, particularly spina bifida. Sodium valproate is regarded as more dangerous than carbamazepine. Benzodiazepines are best avoided in pregnancy, as there is some association with oral cleft defects in newborns, although there is some debate about the magnitude of this risk. Of the atypical antipsychotics there is most experience with olanzapine, although the risk of gestational diabetes may be increased. Of the SSRIs, there is most experience with fluoxetine in pregnancy, although there is an increased risk of premature delivery and reduced birth weight. **[V. pp. 367–72]**

2 **Answer: C.** Dissociative fugue is the diagnosis in this case. Criteria include: a) purposeful travel beyond the usual everyday range, along with b) maintenance of self-care. It also requires c) the criteria of dissociative amnesia to make the diagnosis. These criteria are amnesia, either partial or complete, for recent events that are of a traumatic or stressful nature (which may emerge with collateral history) and the absence of organic brain disorder or excessive fatigue. Stupor requires profound diminution of voluntary movement so is not the diagnosis, likewise amnesia is too general to be the most likely diagnosis. Trance disorder has both loss of personal identity and full awareness of the surroundings. **[I. pp. 154–7]**

3 **Answer: E.** All of these disorders mentioned can cause depression. Other possible organic causes for depression include: various endocrine disorders (such as hyperparathyroidism or Addison's disease), infections (such as infectious mononucleosis), metabolic disorders (such as iron deficiency anaemia or B12/folate deficiency) and neurological causes (e.g. post CVA or multiple sclerosis). **[H. p. 53]**

4 **Answer: E.** Sims defines somatic passivity as: 'a delusional belief that the body is being influenced from outside the self'. It can occur along with somatic hallucinations or real perceptions (as the pain is in this case). Somatic passivity is a first-rank symptom of schizophrenia. While items A, B, D are incorrect, the experience could be said to be item C (a paranoid delusion). However, item E is the term that *closest* fits her experience. **[D. pp. 153–4]**

5 The antidepressant mirtazapine has few anti-muscarinic receptor mediated adverse effects and is thought to have a mechanism of action best described as:

A. Dopamine antagonism.

B. Noradrenergic and specific serotonergic antagonism.

C. Serotonin and noradrenaline reuptake inhibition.

D. Serotonin-dopamine antagonism.

E. Selective serotonin reuptake inhibition.

6 A 35-year-old man with a diagnosis of schizoaffective disorder is referred by his GP for review in the outpatient department. He is on risperidone 6 mg daily, having been recently decreased from 8 mg. He has been noted by the GP to be very restless. At interview he has marked lower limb movement, although he remains seated. He reports that he is sleeping well without a hypnotic. He continues to attend his rehabilitation programme and is receiving good reports from staff. What is the most likely cause of this man's restlessness?

A. Akathisia.   B. Anxiety.

C. Catatonic excitement.   D. Mania.

E. Restless leg syndrome.

7 A 21-year-old woman is convinced that her nose is physically misshapen. Having been reviewed surgically, and found to have no obvious nasal pathology or abnormality, she is referred to you for psychiatric assessment. Which of the following ICD-10 diagnoses is the most likely in this case?

A. Delusional disorder.   B. Hypochondriacal disorder.

C. Panic disorder.   D. Post-traumatic stress disorder.

E. Somatisation disorder.

8 A man with a glass eye can perceive that a cat in the foreground is nearer to him than a tree in the background. Which of the following cues is the most likely one that allows him to perceive this?

A. Accommodation.   B. Convergence.

C. Interposition.   D. Size constancy.

E. Stereopsis.

5 **Answer: B.** Mirtazapine is a noradrenergic and selective serotonin antagonist (NaSSA). Its presynaptic α_2 antagonism at the serotonergic neurone increases its release of serotonin into the synapse. It also is a selective antagonist at several serotonin receptors at the post-synaptic membrane. [**U. p. 70**]

6 **Answer: A.** Akathisia is distinguished from other causes of restlessness by the prominence of lower limb restlessness. Acute akathisia occurs within hours or weeks of starting antipsychotics or after increasing the dose. It also may occur after a reduction in the dose to treat other extra-pyramidal side-effects. Risperidone is one of the atypical antipsychotics most strongly associated with EPSEs. Restless leg syndrome is characterised by subjective experience of restlessness interfering with sleep. [**D. p. 339; V. p. 96; X. p. 167; AK. p. 487**]

7 **Answer: A.** Beliefs in hypochondriacal disorder do not have the same fixity as those in schizophrenic disorders accompanied by somatic delusions. If the patient has this conviction, they should be diagnosed with a delusional disorder. In panic and anxiety disorders, the patients are usually reassured by a physiological explanation. Post-traumatic stress disorder is a distracter. [**I. pp. 164–6**]

8 **Answer: C.** What is being described is depth perception. Since the man has just one functioning eye, he is dependent on monocular cues for depth perception. Convergence, accommodation and stereopsis are binocular cues. Interposition is a monocular cue, and might be used if part of the cat can be seen to be hiding part of the tree trunk, allowing the difference in depth to be perceived. Size constancy is a visual constancy and is not a cue for depth perception. [**C. pp. 361–2**]

9 While doing a physical examination on a patient, you notice that his pupils have irregular margins. They accommodate but are not responsive to light. From the list below, what is the most probable cause for this presentation?

A. Anorexia nervosa.

B. Cocaine abuse.

C. Neurosyphilis.

D. Opiate intoxication.

E. Opiate withdrawal.

10 The parents of a 22-year-old patient who has just been diagnosed with paranoid schizophrenia want to know what the risk of relapse is if their son does not take prophylactic antipsychotic medication. Which answer is correct?

A. 47% risk in a year.

B. 57% risk in a year.

C. 77% risk in a year.

D. 77% risk in two years.

E. 97% risk in a year.

11 A 35-year-old woman with a long history of treatment for schizoaffective disorder is referred for assessment by the obstetrics team. She has just given birth to a healthy baby and wishes to breast feed. They are seeking immediate advice regarding her medication and the risks of breastfeeding. Which of the following medications needs to be most urgently reviewed?

A. Carbamazepine.

B. Diazepam.

C. Fluoxetine.

D. Olanzapine.

E. Sodium valproate.

12 A three-year-old child assumes that his way of thinking is the only way. What term below best describes this phenomenon?

A. Centration.

B. Conservation.

C. Egocentrism.

D. Object permanence.

E. Reversibility.

9   **Answer: C.** This type of presentation is called the Argyll–Robertson pupil, caused by neurosyphilis. In opiate intoxication the pupils are pin-point while in withdrawal they are dilated. There are no specific pupil changes in anorexia nervosa. **[AB. p. 73]**

10   **Answer: B.** From the Crow study the risk of relapse of schizophrenia is 57% in the first year. **[V. p. 57]**

11   **Answer: B.** Repeated doses of long-acting benzodiazepines, such as diazepam, can result in lethargy and weight loss in infants. Carbamazepine is considered low risk in breastfeeding as levels are relatively low in breast milk. Valproate appears relatively safe, although with a small but finite risk of haematological effects in the infant. Adverse effects have not been reported for most fluoxetine-exposed infants. Olanzapine is excreted in breast milk with infants exposed to about 1% of the maternal dose with no adverse effects. **[X. pp. 199–206]**

12   **Answer: C.** Egocentrism occurs in Piaget's pre-operational stage (age two to seven years). Centration occurs at the same stage, where the child often pays attention to only part of a given task. Conservation and reversibility are also part of the pre-operational stage. Object perma-nence occurs in the sensori-motor stage. **[C. pp. 136–7]**

13 A 25-year-old woman presents with depression. Which of the following is least likely to be of aetiological significance?

A. Barbiturates.

B. Oral contraceptive pill.

C. Prolonged amphetamine use.

D. Reserpine.

E. Steroids.

14 A GP refers a 24-year-old man to you for a psychiatric opinion. He believes the patient meets DSM-IV criteria for antisocial personality disorder and lists various features the man has in evidence. Which of the following features that he has listed would most lead you to doubt this diagnosis, based on DSM-IV criteria?

A. Consistent irresponsibility.

B. Deceitfulness.

C. Impulsivity.

D. Irritability.

E. Recurrent suicidal behaviour.

15 You plan to prescribe an antipsychotic to a 45-year-old man with schizophrenia who has type II diabetes. Previously he had gynaecomastia secondary to antipsychotic-mediated hyperprolactinaemia. Which one of the following choices would be most suitable?

A. Aripiprazole.

B. Clozapine.

C. Olanzapine.

D. Risperidone.

E. Sulpiride.

16 Which of the following factors would help to distinguish the presentation of malingering from factitious disorder?

A. Lack of cooperation during the diagnostic evaluation.

B. Lack of cooperation in complying with the prescribed treatment regimen.

C. Marked discrepancy between the person's claimed stress or disability and the objective findings.

D. Medico-legal context to presentation.

E. Presence of antisocial personality disorder.

13 **Answer: B.** Oral contraceptives are no longer considered to cause depression. All the other medications mentioned in the question are recognised causes of depression. **[H. p. 53]**

14 **Answer: E.** The features listed in items A to D are all taken directly from DSM-IV criteria for antisocial personality disorder. 'Recurrent suicidal behaviour', however, is listed as a criterion for borderline personality disorder. There is obviously overlap with the latter and the criterion of 'reckless disregard for safety of self or others' in antisocial personality disorder, but the two are not synonymous criteria. Note that 'impulsivity' is also a criterion for borderline personality disorder, highlighting the fact that many patients will fulfil criteria for more than one personality disorder. **[J. pp. 649–50, 654]**

15 **Answer: A.** Aripiprazole does not cause substantial weight gain and is not associated with impaired glucose tolerance. It also does not cause hyperprolactinaemia. Clozapine, olanzapine and risperidone are associated with impaired glucose tolerance and should be avoided in this group. Risperidone and sulpiride cause significant hyperprolactinaemia. **[Q. pp. 192–5; V. pp. 20–3]**

16 **Answer: D.** Malingering differs from factitious disorder in that the motivation for the presentation in malingering is an external incentive, while in factitious disorder external incentives are absent. Factitious disorder would be suggested by evidence of an intrapsychic need to maintain the sick role. **[AH. pp. 309–10]**

17 A 56-year-old male patient with a 30-year history of paranoid schizophrenia attends your psychiatric clinic. His family have noted that he is able to hold his head several inches above his pillow while lying on his bed. The term that closest fits his experience is?

A. Mannerism.

B. Perseveration.

C. Stereotypy.

D. Torticollis.

E. Waxy flexibility.

18 Which of the following DSM-IV personality disorders is more frequently diagnosed in men?

A. Avoidant personality disorder.

B. Borderline personality disorder.

C. Dependent personality disorder.

D. Histrionic personality disorder.

E. Schizoid personality disorder.

19 A patient on the psychiatric ward took an overdose; you are called to review the patient. When you arrive at the scene, you see the patient lying in the bed with eyes closed. You call his name: he opens his eyes and answers the question with inappropriate words. There are no spontaneous movements on request but he is able to push away your hand when you pinch his skin. What is the Glasgow Coma Scale score for this patient?

A. 9

B. 10.

C. 11

D. 12.

E. 13.

20 You wish to prescribe an antidepressant for an 80-year-old man who suffers from closed-angle glaucoma, and has a history of duodenal ulcers. He also complains of restless unsatisfactory sleep and poor appetite leading to weight loss. Which one of these medications is the most suitable?

A. Amitriptyline.

B. Escitalopram.

C. Mirtazapine.

D. Sertraline.

E. Venlafaxine.

17   **Answer: E.** 'Psychological pillow' is the term for what is occuring in this case. The phenomenon described is waxy flexibility, where a patient's limbs can be placed in a position in which they remain. Mannerisms are repetitive voluntary purposeful movements, whereas stereotypes are repetitive purposeless movements carried out in a uniform way. Torticollis is characterised by involuntary tonic contractions or intermittent spasms of neck muscles, and can occur in tardive dyskinesia. **[A. p. 250]**

18   **Answer: E.** Borderline, dependent and histrionic personality disorders are diagnosed more frequently in women. Avoidant personality disorder has a roughly equal sex incidence. Antisocial, narcissistic and schizoid personality disorders are diagnosed more frequently in males. Some of these differences may reflect true sex differences rather than differential diagnostic patterns. **[J. pp. 631–2, 639, 663]**

19   **Answer: C.** There are three components to a Glasgow Coma Scale score (maximum scores in brackets): best eye response (4), best verbal response (5), and best motor response (6). The Glasgow Coma Scale is scored between 3 and 15 with 3 being the worst score. **[www.unc. edu/~rowlett/units/scales/glasgow.htm]**

20   **Answer: C.** Amitriptyline exacerbates closed-angle glaucoma. Sertraline and escitalopram are both SSRIs which are associated with GIT bleeds. Venlafaxine may exacerbate insomnia and anorexia. **[Q. pp. 202, 208, 210]**

21 A 20-year-old woman presents to the Casualty department having inflicted superficial cuts to her wrists. While waiting to be seen she became belligerent and verbally aggressive with staff. She reports that she has harmed herself on several occasions previously. She describes recent paranoid ideation, and says that she has begun binge eating again in recent months. The current episode of self-harm was precipitated by a row with her boyfriend of three weeks, who she describes as the 'love of my life'. There is a history of unstable employment and relationships. According to DSM-IV criteria, which is the most likely diagnosis?

A. Antisocial personality disorder.

B. Borderline personality disorder.

C. Dependent personality disorder.

D. Histrionic personality disorder.

E. Paranoid personality disorder.

22 Which of the following figures was most vocal in the criticism of psychiatry as an agent of social control?

A. Goffman.   B. Mechanic.

C. Parsons.   D. Wing.

E. Szasz.

23 Which of the following authors is least associated with having made major contributions to the understanding of depression?

A. Andreasen.   B. Beck.

C. Brown and Harris.   D. Seligman.

E. Wolpe.

24 A 68-year-old man who has suffered a cerebrovascular accident is suspected of having a pseudobulbar palsy. Which of the following findings would lead you to doubt this?

A. Brisk jaw jerk.   B. Ischaemic heart disease.

C. Labile emotions.   D. Nasal speech.

E. Spastic tongue.

21 **Answer: B.** This woman demonstrates the following features of border-line personality disorder:

- A pattern of unstable and intense interpersonal relationships.
- Recurrent suicidal behaviour, gestures, or threats, or self-mutilating behaviour.
- Transient stress-related paranoid ideation.
- Impulsivity as characterised by her binge eating and substance abuse.
- Inappropriate, intense anger or difficulty controlling anger.

She may demonstrate traits of other Cluster B personality disorders, for example:

- Antisocial personality disorder: impulsivity or failure to plan ahead, irritability and aggressiveness.
- Histrionic personality disorder: considers relationships to be more intimate than they actually are, shows self-dramatisation and exaggerated expression of emotion. **[AH. pp. 291–3]**

22 **Answer: E.** Thomas Szasz was part of the anti-psychiatry movement, who viewed mental illness as a myth and saw the role of the psychiatrist as an agent of social control. Parsons described the social role of doctors and the sick role. Mechanic described illness behaviour. Wing described secondary handicap. Goffman described total institutions. **[G. pp. 71–2, 77–9]**

23 **Answer: A.** Nancy Andreasen has mainly contributed to the neurobiological understanding of schizophrenia. Wolpe viewed depression as a conditioned response following repeated losses in the past. Seligman postulated learned helplessness as a consequence of repeated exposure to uncontrollable traumas, which can be complicated by depression. Beck, on the other the hand, described the cognitive aspects of depression. Brown and Harris described high rates of depression among inner-city London lower socioeconomic group females and suggested some vulnerability factors which predispose to depression. **[H. p. 54]**

24 **Answer: D.** Lower motor neuron lesions (bulbar palsy) are associated with nasal speech, flaccid tongue, normal/absent jaw jerk and normal emotions. Answers A, C and E are associated with upper motor neuron lesions (pseudobulbar palsy). Pseudobulbar palsy can be caused by cerebrovascular accidents or demyelination, while bulbar palsy can be caused by infections or syringobulbia. **[F. p. 109]**

25 Goffman described several reactions to the mortification process. Which one of the following means 'the patient pretends to show acceptance'?

A. Betrayal funnel.

B. Colonisation.

C. Conversion.

D. Institutionalisation.

E. Withdrawal.

26 A 22-year-old man is sent for assessment by his GP for depression which is not responding to antidepressant therapy. During the course of the interview, the man reports that from childhood he has wanted to be a girl. He frequently dresses and goes out in public in female clothing. He reports that he is sexually attracted to men, which he believes is evidence of the wrong gender assignment. He has no paraphilic interests. What is the most likely diagnosis?

A. Egodystonic sexual orientation.

B. Fetishism.

C. Gender identity disorder.

D. Polymorphously perverse.

E. Transvestic fetishism.

27 In 1920 Watson and Rayner used a classical conditioning model with Little Albert (11 months old) who then developed a white rat phobia. He subsequently developed a phobia of any furry animal. Which of the terms below best describes this new phobia of furry animals?

A. Generalisation.

B. Higher order conditioning.

C. Incubation.

D. Spontaneous recovery.

E. Trace conditioning.

28 A 23-year-old Irish man is referred for assessment after displaying a number of psychotic symptoms. His GP suspects he has schizophrenia. Which of the following psychotic symptoms would most lead you to suspect the diagnosis is indeed schizophrenia?

A. He believes he has been given special powers to heal people.

B. He believes that aliens from Neptune have removed his brain and that his hollow cranium now allows everyone in his vicinity to hear his thoughts.

C. He believes that US Secretary of State Hillary Clinton is in love with him from the way she looks at him from the TV.

D. He believes the IRA is plotting to blow up his garden shed.

E. He hears his own thoughts being spoken aloud a few seconds after he has had the thought.

25 **Answer B.** Betrayal funnel is a concept referring to the sending of a patient to hospital by relatives. The others are all possible reactions to the mortification process. **[R. p. 142]**

26 **Answer: C.** Gender identity disorder is characterised by a strong and persistent cross-gender identification characterised by the stated desire to be the other sex, frequent passing as the other sex and a desire to live or be treated as the other sex. In egodystonic sexual orientation the patient states that the sustained pattern of homosexual arousal is unwanted and is a source of distress. There is a desire to acquire heterosexual orientation. Fetishism involves sexual arousal to non-living objects and is a type of paraphilia. Polymorphous perversion is the harbouring of more than one form of paraphilia. **[AH. pp. 259–61; D. pp. 251–3]**

27 **Answer: A.** Generalisation is the classical conditioning term that best describes this fear of furry animals. Higher order conditioning is learning a new conditioned stimulus through association with the original conditioned stimulus (which now becomes the unconditioned stimulus). Incubation results from repeated brief exposure to the conditioned stimulus and causes an increase in strength of the conditioned response. **[F. p. 2]**

28 **Answer: B.** The main difficulty in this question is determining whether answer B or E is the more correct. Answers A, C and D are examples of grandiose or paranoid delusions and could easily be seen in a manic episode. B and E, however, contain first-rank symptoms of schizophrenia. B is probably more correct, though, as apart from being the first rank symptom of thought broadcasting, it is also a bizarre delusion (culturally inappropriate and completely impossible) which is mentioned in both ICD-10 and DSM-IV as having diagnostic significance. **[I. pp. 87–8]**

29 On physical examination, you notice that a patient has coarse tremor whenever he attempts to grasp something, but you cannot see these tremors when he is sitting in a relaxed state. What is the most possible cause for his tremors?

A. Alcohol abuse.

B. Anxiety.

C. Cerebellar disease.

D. Lithium treatment.

E. Long-term antipsychotic depot injection.

30 The resolution of Erikson's stage of Identity versus Role Confusion gives rise to which one of the following terms?

A. Care.

B. Competence.

C. Fidelity.

D. Hope.

E. Wisdom.

31 A 65-year-old single man presents with a history of alcohol dependence syndrome. He recently relapsed and has been drinking approximately 20 units of alcohol per day for the past two months. He has not had a drink in 24 hours. He has a history of seizures on one previous occasion when withdrawing from alcohol. Which of the following is the most appropriate approach to his management?

A. Inpatient detoxification with chlordiazepoxide, carbamazepine and parenteral thiamine.

B. Inpatient detoxification with chlordiazepoxide and parenteral thiamine.

C. Outpatient detoxification with chlordiazepoxide.

D. Outpatient detoxification with chlordiazepoxide and carbamazepine.

E. Outpatient detoxification with chlordiazepoxide, carbamazepine and oral thiamine.

32 A gambler playing the slot machines is displaying which type of partial reinforcement?

A. Constant interval.

B. Fixed interval.

C. Fixed ratio.

D. Variable interval.

E. Variable ratio.

29 **Answer: C.** Cerebellar disease causes intentional tremor. All the other options given cause resting tremor. **[AB. p. 73]**

30 **Answer: C.** Erikson postulated a genetically determined sequence of psychosocial stages or crises. Each arises from conflict between two conflicting personality outcomes, one adaptive, one maladaptive. Identity versus Role Confusion occurs in adolescence. **[T. p. 57]**

31 **Answer: B.** Elderly patients with a history of withdrawal seizures should be detoxified as inpatients. All inpatient detoxification regimes should include prophylactic parenteral thiamine for Wernicke's encephalopathy as there is limited evidence for oral thiamine. There is no definitive evidence for the use of anticonvulsants for alcohol withdrawal. **[V. pp. 304, 313, 314]**

32 **Answer: E.** Variable ratio reinforcement produces a relatively constant rate of response, and is the type of reinforcement seen in gambling behaviour. Constant interval is a distracter. **[F. p. 3]**

33 Which of the following is not a predictor of poor outcome in cases of depression?

A. Comorbid alcohol use.

B. Comorbid dysthymia.

C. Comorbid personality disorder.

D. Late onset.

E. Severe symptoms at index episode.

34 DSM-IV uses a multiaxial assessment system. Of the following pairings, choose the one which most correctly describes an axis used by DSM-IV:

A. Axis I: General Medical Condition.

B. Axis II: Mental Retardation.

C. Axis III: Psychosocial and Environmental Problems.

D. Axis IV: Clinical Disorder.

E. Axis V: Global Assessment of Coping.

35 Bandura's Social Learning theory postulates that learning occurs following observation and imitation. Which one of the following terms is not associated with this theory?

A. Attentional processes.

B. Motor reproduction.

C. Reinforcement.

D. Resolution.

E. Retention.

36 A 19-year-old man presents to Casualty seeking detoxification from benzodiazepines. He reports that he has been taking diazepam 15 mg daily. He says that he has not taken any in 48 hours and says that he is experiencing withdrawal symptoms. Which of the following symptoms is he most likely to describe?

A. Anxiety symptoms.

B. Decreased consciousness.

C. Extreme fatigue.

D. Runny nose and eyes.

E. Vomiting.

33 **Answer: D.** Early onset of depression is a predictor of poor outcome along with the other items from the question. **[H. p. 55]**

34 **Answer: B.** It is important to be familiar with DSM-IV as well as ICD-10 for the exams. Axis II is used to list both personality disorders and mental retardation. Axis V is the Global Assessment of *Functioning*. The other correct pairings are: Axis 1: Clinical Disorders, Axis III: General Medical Conditions and Axis IV: Psychosocial and Environmental Problems. **[J. p. 25]**

35 **Answer: D.** The order of the processes are: attentional processes, retention and memory permanence using rehearsal, motor reproduction and reinforcement. Resolution is not a component. **[T. p. 56]**

36 **Answer: A.** Extreme fatigue is more characteristic of withdrawal from amphetamines. Decreased consciousness is more characteristic of withdrawal from cocaine. Runny nose and eyes (rhinitis) is more characteristic of withdrawal from heroin. Vomiting is more characteristic of withdrawal from alcohol or barbiturates. **[V. p. 346]**

37 The 'cocktail party' effect of being able to hear your name being mentioned elsewhere in the room, while you are talking to someone else, is best described by which of the terms below?

A. Automatic attention.
B. Controlled attention.
C. Divided attention.
D. Selective attention.
E. Sustained attention.

38 In an experiment, a boy learns a list of words in a green room. He then is asked to recall this list in another green room. He is then brought back to the first green room and asked to learn a second list of words. He is brought to a red room and asked to recall this list. He scores better when the recall room was the same colour as the memorisation room. The experiment is repeated, so that he recalls in the red room first, then in a green room. He still scores better when the recall room was the same colour as the memorisation room. Which of the following terms most closely describes the psychological phenomenon being described in terms of his poorer scores in the red room?

A. Context-dependent forgetting.

B. Cue-dependent forgetting.

C. Proactive interference.

D. Retroactive interference.

E. State-dependent forgetting.

39 A 70-year-old female patient who has had memory problems for the last few months has started getting agitated because she can see people coming to her room and disturbing her. On examination, you find bradykinesia, limb rigidity and gait disturbances. Her Mini-Mental State Examination score is 18/30. Which of the following medications is best avoided?

A. Fluoxetine.
B. Clonazepam.
C. Memantine.
D. Olanzapine.
E. Carbamazepine.

40 According to Chess and Thomas in the New York Longitudinal Study, children have nine categories of temperament. Which of the following is not one of them?

A. Activity.
B. Adaptation to change.
C. Distractibility.
D. Rhythmicity.
E. Temerity.

37 **Answer: D.** Selective (focused) attention best describes this: dichotic listening studies show that alternative information is processed simultaneously and can be attended to if required. With automatic attention, proficiency reduces the necessary conscious effort required. With sustained attention performance progressively deteriorates. Controlled attention requires effort. **[F. pp. 7–8]**

38 **Answer: A.** It seems being in a similarly coloured room helps his recall, thus it is acting as a cue. *Cue-dependent forgetting* was coined by Tulving to cover both *context-dependent forgetting* and *state-dependent forgetting*. *Context-dependent forgetting* refers to external (environment) cues and so is the most appropriate (closest) term. **[O. p. 25]**

39 **Answer: D.** This is a presentation of dementia with Lewy bodies. Antipsychotic medication is best avoided because it can cause worsening of agitation. Approximately 60% of the patients are sensitive to antipsychotics. There is no clear evidence for antidepressants, anticonvulsants or benzodiazepines causing such reaction. The treatment is mostly behavioural and supportive. **[AB. pp. 140–1]**

40 **Answer E.** Temerity is not one of the dimensions. **[R. p. 69]**

41 A 46-year-old married man with a history of dysthymia and who is being treated with an antidepressant presents in the outpatient department complaining of impotence. Which of the following medications is the most likely cause of this problem?

A. Clomipramine.

B. Mirtazapine.

C. Phenelzine.

D. Reboxetine.

E. Venlafaxine.

42 From social psychology theory on interpersonal attraction, having a preference for a relationship which offers the greatest gains with the least expense is described best by which of the following terms?

A. Balance theory.

B. Equity theory.

C. Exchange theory.

D. Proxemics.

E. Similarity hypothesis.

43 Regarding causes and prognosis of mood disorder, which of the following is incorrect?

A. At least 50% of depressed patients recover by six months.

B. At least 50% with depression in remission will have subsequent episodes.

C. Depressive and manic episodes tend to remit spontaneously.

D. Inter-episode intervals tend to shorten over time.

E. Kraepelin viewed manic-depressive illness to be of poor outcome.

44 The following defence mechanisms are considered to be mature defences except:

A. Altruism.

B. Anticipation.

C. Intellectualisation.

D. Sublimation.

E. Suppression.

41 **Answer: E.** The approximate prevalences of sexual side-effects with antidepressants are as follows:

- Tricyclic antidepressants   30%
- Reboxetine   5–10%
- Mirtazapine   25%
- MAOIs   40%
- Venlafaxine   70%.

[V. p. 232]

42 **Answer: C.** This is best described by exchange theory. Equity theory describes that the relationship should be fair with equal gains to both parties in the longer term. Proxemics describes interpersonal space. Similarity or matching hypothesis describes the pairing of individuals to form romantic partners, i.e. they are closely matched regarding mutual rewards. Balance theory is a distracter. [F. p. 20]

43 **Answer: E.** Kraepelin viewed manic-depressive insanity to be of good outcome. However, this is now questioned. All other statements are correct. [H. p. 55; M. p. 721]

44 **Answer: C.** Intellectualisation is considered to be a neurotic defence mechanism as it involves overly using intellectual processes to avoid conflict. Other defence mechanisms considered to be 'mature' are asceticism and humour. It should be noted that various psychoanalytic authors have differing views on how the defence mechanisms should be classified. [P. p. 585]

45 The Gestalt laws of perception explain that humans perceive whole figures and therefore in situations where there are two possible figures, we
will alternate between perceiving each one. However, we cannot perceive
both at the same time. The following are Gestalt grouping principles
except:

    A. Closure.
        B. Continuation.

    C. Construction.
       D. Proximity.

    E. Similarity.

46 A 25-year-old woman with a diagnosis of depression is reviewed in the
outpatient department. She anxiously describes the experience of hearing voices at night in bed while she goes to sleep. Which of the following
perceptual abnormalities is this woman experiencing?

    A. Extracampine hallucinations.
    B. Hypnagogic hallucinations.

    C. Hypnopompic hallucinations.
    D. Pseudohallucinations.

    E. Reflex hallucinations.

47 Which of the intelligence quotient (IQ) tests described below can be
used earliest (at the youngest age) to measure IQ in humans?

    A. National Adult Reading Test (NART).

    B. Stanford–Binet Intelligence Scale.

    C. Wechsler Adult Intelligence Scale (WAIS).

    D. Wechsler Intelligence Scale for Children-Revised (WISC-R).

    E. Wechsler Pre-school and Primary School Intelligence scale
(WPPSI).

48 From a psychotherapy ethical viewpoint, which of the following appears
to be the least objectionable practice by a psychotherapist?

    A. The clinician accepts a cup of coffee bought by a paranoid patient
who has only just started to trust him.

    B. The clinician attempts to equalise the relationship by spending
most of the session talking about his own family difficulties, thereby
showing the patient she is not alone in having problems.

    C. The clinician drives the patient home so he can continue extra
sessional work during the drive.

    D. The clinician hugs the patient while she recounts tearfully episodes
of her childhood abuse by her father.

    E. The clinician suspects he has a pilonidal sinus and asks the patient
to have a look.

45 **Answer: C.** The Gestalt laws of perception describe grouping principles of Closure, Continuation, Proximity and Similarity. Construction is not one of them. **[O. pp. 210–11]**

46 **Answer: B.** Hypnagogic hallucinations occur while going asleep. Hypnopompic hallucinations occur on waking. Sims (1995) comments that the importance of these phenomena is to recognise their existence and to realise that they are not necessarily abnormal, although they may be truly hallucinatory. Reflex hallucinations occur when a stimulus in one modality produces a hallucination in another. A pseudohallucination is a perceptual experience which is figurative, not concretely real, and occurs in inner subjective space not in external objective space. Extracampine hallucinations are experienced by the patient as outside the limits of the sensory field. **[D. p. 96]**

47 **Answer: B.** The Stanford–Binet measures from age two years, WPPSI from four to six and a half years and the WISC from five to 15 years of age. Slap yourself if you chose the NART. **[F. pp. 40–1]**

48 **Answer: A.** Gabbard distinguishes *boundary violations* from *boundary crossings*. Boundary violations may be sexual or non-sexual (as are most of the violations presented here). While the situations presented are sparse in details, the clinician who accepts a small present from a patient who would be hurt/paranoid at its refusal could be seen as a boundary crossing as it may be ultimately therapeutically constructive. Context is of course important: it may be appropriate to hug a patient back if for example she hugs you after telling you that her mother has just died (as opposed to shoving her away and calling for security). However, physical contact is to be avoided in the vulnerable patient. The situation in option C is a boundary violation as it is breaking agreed limits on the timing of sessions. Self-disclosure is problematic if it is excessive and/or if it burdens the patient with the therapist's problems. Apart from the small matter of criminal indecent exposure, the situation in E could also be seen as burdening the patient with the therapist's problems. **[AM. pp. 141–60]**

49 A patient has Wernicke's encephalopathy following a history of prolonged alcohol intake. From the list given below, which symptom is unlikely to be seen at this stage?

A. Acute confusional state.   B. Ataxia.

C. Confabulation.   D. Nystagmus.

E. Ophthalmoplegia.

50 The model of attention known as the 'late selection model' was proposed by which one of the following researchers?

A. Broadbent.   B. Cherry.

C. Deutsch-Norman.   D. Kahneman.

E. Treissman.

51 A 45-year-old woman presents as a new patient for assessment. She describes a long history of anxiety when out in public. She recalls the onset of her difficulties when she was 20 and experienced her first panic attack. She avoids social events and in recent times is leaving her home much less frequently. She says that she is fearful of experiencing a panic attack away from home, although she has not had a panic attack in over three months. Which is the most likely diagnosis in this case according to DSM-IV criteria?

A. Agoraphobia with a history of panic disorder.

B. Generalised anxiety disorder.

C. Panic disorder with agoraphobia.

D. Separation anxiety disorder.

E. Social phobia.

52 Which of the following terms is not related to Goffman's description of institutionalisation?

A. Betrayal funnel.   B. Batch living.

C. Binary living.   D. Institutional neurosis.

E. Role stripping.

49 **Answer: C.** Confabulation is present in Korsakoff's psychosis while Wernicke's encephalopathy is a classical tetrad of symptoms (ataxia, ophthalmoplegia, nystagmus and acute confusional state) caused by thiamine deficiency and which is related to alcohol abuse. **[AB. p. 148]**

50 **Answer: C.** The late selection model was proposed by Deutsch-Norman and rejected Broadbent's claim that information is filtered out early on. Their theory postulates that all information is analysed before selecting pertinent material for selective attention. **[O. pp. 185–7]**

51 **Answer: C.** DSM-IV classifies the following disorders:

- panic disorder without agoraphobia
- panic disorder with agoraphobia
- agoraphobia without a history of panic disorder.

Agoraphobia is not a code-able disorder, and so there is no diagnosis of agoraphobia with panic disorder. Therefore this woman has panic disorder with agoraphobia. Her avoidance of public situations is provoked by the fear of a panic attack rather than a fear of social performance which would characterise a social phobia. In generalised anxiety disorder there is excessive anxiety and worry occurring more days than not for at least six months. The focus of the anxiety is not confined to features of an Axis I disorder, e.g. the anxiety or worry is not about having a panic attack. Separation anxiety disorder has an onset before the age of 18 years. **[AH. pp. 77, 209–16]**

52 **Answer: D.** Institutional neurosis was described by Barton as symptoms of submissiveness, apathy, diminished self-esteem, and inability to plan, along with symptoms of withdrawal. Withdrawal was also described by Goffman as a reaction to the mortification process. **[F. pp. 65–6]**

53 Which of the following is not known to be a complication of anorexia nervosa?

A. Hypocalcaemia.

B. Hypoglycaemia.

C. Hypokalaemia.

D. Hypomagnesaemia.

E. Reduced plasma amylase.

54 Which of the following situations in which patient confidentiality has been breached may be most defensible ethically?

A. A consultant psychiatrist warns a consultant oncologist that it may be best not to have a meeting with a certain patient as the patient blames the oncologist for her husband's death and has thought of punching him.

B. A police officer wishes to know by telephone if a man they have detained has a history of drug abuse. The psychiatric SHO confirms this after the police officer assures her that the information is 'off the record'.

C. A psychiatric registrar is worried about a patient she saw in clinic who has thoughts of self-harm and confides in her husband.

D. A psychiatric SHO presents a case conference to colleagues within the same hospital without having got consent from the patient.

E. The secretary of the community mental health team shares a funny story she heard during dictation with her colleagues about a local patient who was caught in bed with a woman by the woman's husband.

55 Baddeley and Hitch proposed a 'Working Memory Model' to explain human memory in a functional manner. Which of the following is not a component of this model?

A. A network of nodes.

B. Articulatory loop.

C. Central executive.

D. Primary acoustic store.

E. Visuospatial scratchpad.

56 Which of the following syndromes is not associated with a psychotic illness?

A. Couvade syndrome.

B. De Clerambault's syndrome.

C. Fregoli syndrome.

D. Othello syndrome.

E. Syndrome of subjective doubles.

53 **Answer: E.** Plasma amylase levels, like cholesterol levels, tend to be raised in anorexia nervosa. **[H. p. 95]**

54 **Answer: A.** All of the scenarios involve breaches of confidentiality. Scenarios C, D and E are probably common and are especially serious if the patient can be identified. Situations where police officers are looking for information which could be prejudicial to the patient must always be treated with caution: the reasons for provision of information must be explicit and advice should be sought from colleagues, including legal advice in some circumstances. Since the Tarasoff ruling, psychiatrists have a duty to warn others where they perceive a material risk to others: even in this situation it is important to try to involve patients in the process, for example by warning patients how their statements may lead to a situation whereby the confidentiality will have to be breached. **[AM. pp. 105–40]**

55 **Answer A.** Baddeley and Hitch's 'Working Memory Model' described three modality based stores (the Articulatory Loop, the Visuospatial Scratchpad and the Primary Acoustic Store) and a limited capacity modality free Central Executive. The Node Network is associated with the hierarchical network model of Collins and Quillian. **[O. pp. 253–5]**

56 **Answer: A.** In Couvade syndrome a person develops extreme anxiety and various physical symptoms of pregnancy when his partner is pregnant. He may have morning sickness, abdominal pains, constipation, food craving etc. It is thought to be a manifestation of anxiety. It may be an expression of frustrated creativity, jealousy of the attention paid to the pregnant partner or over-identification with the pregnant partner. It is usually managed with reassurance. In Fregoli syndrome the patient believes that ordinary people in his environment are persecutors in disguise. In De Clerambault's syndrome the patient believes that another person loves him intensely. The object of the delusion is often of higher social status. Othello syndrome involves delusion of infidelity on the part of a sexual partner. In the syndrome of subjective doubles the patient believes that doubles of himself exist. **[H. pp. 160–3]**

57 Which of the terms below best describes a type of perseveration involving repetition of the last word's last syllable?

A. Alogia.

B. Echologia.

C. Echolalia.

D. Logoclonia.

E. Logorrhoea.

58 A psychiatrist is asked to see a 60-year-old man with terminal cancer who is suspected of being depressed. The patient has had severe pain and is being treated with high-dose morphine. She is concerned to note that there appears to be respiratory depression. She communicates her concern that this respiratory depression may hasten the patient's death to the oncologist: he agrees this may well happen but believes the treatment is justified. Which of the following ethics terms is the oncologist most likely to use to justify his treatment?

A. Deontology.

B. Double effect.

C. Moral absolutism.

D. Paternalism.

E. Utilitarianism.

59 Albert was recently involved in a car accident that resulted in memory loss for a short period of time. Which of the following is the best predictor of his prognosis?

A. Anterograde amnesia.

B. Post-traumatic amnesia.

C. Psychogenic fugue.

D. Retrograde amnesia.

E. Transient global amnesia.

60 Maslow's hierarchy of needs can be represented by a pyramid. Which of the following statements is true of this pyramid?

A. Aesthetic needs are higher than self-actualisation.

B. Cognitive needs are higher than esteem needs.

C. Cognitive needs are higher than aesthetic needs.

D. The need for competence is lower than esteem needs.

E. The need for love and belongingness is higher than esteem needs.

57 **Answer: D.** Logoclonia is the term. Logorrhoea describes voluble garrulous speech. Echolalia is the automatic imitation and repetition of another person's speech or words. Echologia is repetition of another individual's speech using one's own words or phrases. Alogia is poverty of speech, with responses being often limited to single words. **[F. pp. 80–1]**

58 **Answer: B.** The doctrine of double effect makes a distinction between the intended good effect (wishing to relieve the severe pain) and the unintended, albeit foreseen, bad effect (causing the patient's death). Deontology is an ethical approach that seeks rules or duties to inform ethical decision making, while utilitarianism seeks to produce the greatest good for the greatest number of people. Moral absolutism refers to having absolute rules that govern moral decisions, e.g. one can never lie. Paternalism in medicine has been described as the 'doctor knows best' model, but has been refined by distinguishing *strong* and *weak* forms of paternalism. **[AN. pp. 61–2, 74–5, 239–40]**

59 **Answer: B.** Post-traumatic amnesia is a loss of memory for the period of the head injury and the period following it (until normal memory resumes). It is the best predictor of prognosis compared to other types of amnesia. Transient global amnesia is a syndrome of amnesia lasting 6–24 hours and is caused by transient ischaemic changes of the temporal lobe. Psychogenic fugue is a distracter in this question. **[AB. p. 154]**

60 **Answer B.** Moving from higher to more basic needs, the order of needs is: Self-actualisation, Aesthetic needs, Cognitive needs, Esteem needs (includes competence), Love and Belongingness, Safety needs, Physiological needs. **[T. p. 77]**

61 A 65-year-old right-handed man is seen in hospital following a cerebrovascular accident. At interview he is noted to have significant difficulties with comprehension. He is also noted to speak fluently but with numerous errors in the use of words, syntax and grammar. Which of the following best describes the location of the cortical lesion in this man's case?

A. Left angular gyrus.

B. Left premotor cortex.

C. Left temporal lobe.

D. Right frontal lobe.

E. Right temporal lobe.

62 Which of the following terms is not part of Schneider's classification of thought disorder?

A. Desultory.

B. Drivelling.

C. Fusion.

D. Omission.

E. Overinclusion.

63 According to Masters and Johnson's phases of response cycle of human sexuality, all of the following are main phases except:

A. Arousal.

B. Desire.

C. Orgasm.

D. Plateau.

E. Satisfaction.

64 Each of the following is one of the commonly accepted 'four principles' of bioethical practice, except:

A. Beneficence.

B. Confidentiality.

C. Justice.

D. Nonmaleficence.

E. Respect for autonomy.

61 **Answer: A.** This man has Wernicke's dysphasia (sensory or receptive dysphasia), resulting from a lesion to the angular gyrus in the posterior part of the superior gyrus of the dominant temporal lobe. Broca's dysphasia (expressive or motor dysphasia) results from a lesion to the precentral gyrus in the dominant frontal cortex. In 90% of right-handed people the left hemisphere plays the predominant role in speech. Wernicke's dysphasia can be distinguished from Broca's dysphasia by the fluency of speech. **[D. pp. 159–63]**

62 **Answer: E.** Overinclusion, an inability to circumscribe a problem or maintain meaningful boundaries, was described by Cameron as part of his classification of thought disorder. **[F. pp. 80–1]**

63 **Answer: E.** The phases of response cycle of human sexuality according to Masters and Johnson (1966) are the following: desire, arousal, plateau, orgasm and resolution. Satisfaction is not one of them. **[H. p. 103]**

64 **Answer: B.** Beauchamps and Childress are associated with the four principles. Beneficence refers to doing good while nonmaleficence refers to avoiding harm. Respect for autonomy means we must respect the wishes of persons with capacity, and justice ensures we consider fairness in providing benefits. Respect for confidentiality is of course important in ethical practice but comes under some of the four principles such as respect for autonomy. **[AM. pp. 33–9]**

65 The theory of emotion which hypothesises that a stimulus is processed by the thalamus which then sends simultaneous signals to the cortex (conscious experience of emotion) and to the hypothalamus (physiological response) is known as:

A. Cannon-Bard theory.

B. Cognitive appraisal.

C. Cognitive labelling theory.

D. Drive reduction theory.

E. James-Lang theory.

66 A 35-year-old man with schizoaffective disorder presents with urinary retention. Which of the following medications is most likely to be responsible?

A. Carbamazepine.

B. Clomipramine.

C. Clonazepam.

D. Haloperidol decanoate.

E. Lithium.

67 A 43-year-old patient is referred to you for psychiatric assessment with a belief that he sees his wife when he looks at various strangers walking down the street. Which of the following best describes this man's description?

A. Capgras' syndrome.

B. Intermetamorphosis

C. Sosia illusion.

D. Subjective doubles.

E. Fregoli syndrome.

68 Select a term from the following that is one of Allport's stages of discrimination:

A. Bias.

B. Circumlocution.

C. Extermination.

D. Prejudice.

E. Stereotyping.

65 **Answer: A.** This is the Cannon-Bard Theory. Cognitive labelling and appraisal theories suggest that stimuli are evaluated at a cognitive level with simultaneous physiological arousal. Drive reduction is a theory to explain motivation rather than emotion. The James-Lang theory describes how emotions are a result of physiological arousal. [**O. pp. 135, 138**]

66 **Answer: B.** Urinary retention is an anticholinergic side-effect. Clomipramine is one of the most potent anticholinergic medications. Lithium is more likely to cause polyuria. Haloperidol decanoate can cause anticholinergic side-effects but has less potential than clomipramine. Benzodiazepines are not uncommonly used postoperatively to reduce urinary retention. There are isolated case reports of urinary retention with carbamazepine but this is not a common side-effect. [**X. pp. 162, 166, 217**]

67 **Answer: E.** Fregoli syndrome describes where a familiar person (his wife) is falsely identified in strangers. This is in contrast to Capgras' syndrome (where the familiar person is supplanted by a stranger who is their exact double). Sosia illusion describes where, along with the spouse in Capgras, other people have been replaced with doubles. Intermetamorphosis is where the exchange of individuals is reciprocal, with the process involving physical and psychological characteristics. Subjective doubles involve the double of oneself, i.e. a person believes that another individual has been transformed into his own self. [**F. p. 85**]

68 **Answer: C.** Allport's (1954) stages of discrimination are (in order): antilocution (verbal attacks), avoidance, discrimination, physical attack and extermination. The Holocaust is an example of the last. [**C. p. 223**]

69 If a patient is suffering from schizophrenia, which of the following activities of different neurotransmitters is most likely present?

A. Decreased dopaminergic activity.

B. Increased glutamate activity.

C. Decreased alpha-adrenergic activity.

D. Decreased serotonin activity.

E. Decreased glutamate activity.

70 People often attribute their own behaviour to be due to external events but attribute others' behaviour to be due to internal events. This is best described as:

A. Actor-observer bias.

B. Attributional bias.

C. Cognitive dissonance.

D. Fundamental attribution error.

E. Self-serving bias.

71 An advertising company is planning a campaign for an alcoholic beverage. The television advertisement shows a tropical beach. Two actors then walk along the sand drinking the alcoholic beverage. What type of conditioning is the advertising company using in this advertising campaign?

A. Backward conditioning.

B. Higher order conditioning.

C. Simultaneous conditioning

D. Stimulus generalisation.

E. Trace conditioning.

72 A 52-year-old male patient within 48 hours of hospital admission for orthopaedic surgery describes to nursing staff seeing little men walking around his bed. Which of the terms below best describes his symptoms?

A. Autoscopic hallucinations.

B. Extracampine hallucinations.

C. Hypnagogic hallucinations.

D. Lilliputian hallucinations.

E. Pseudohallucinations.

69 **Answer: E.** Glutamate and gamma-aminobutyric acid (GABA) transmitters are reported as hypo-functioning in schizophrenia. Serotonin, dopamine and alpha-adrenaline neurotransmitters have been reported to be overactive. **[AB. p. 182]**

70 **Answer: A.** This is actor-observer bias which is a form of attributional bias. Cognitive dissonance is a theory of attitudinal change. Fundamental attribution error is attributing others' behaviour to internal factors (disposition). Self-serving bias is attributing one's successes to internal factors and one's failings to external factors. **[O. pp. 345–6]**

71 **Answer: A.** Backward conditioning involves the introduction of the conditioned stimulus (CS, the drink) after the unconditioned stimulus (UCS, the tropical beach).

- Trace conditioning: the CS is presented and removed before the UCS so only a memory of the CS remains.
- Simultaneous conditioning: the CS and the UCS are presented together.
- Stimulus generalisation: two similar CS can generate the same conditioned response (CR).
- Higher order conditioning: the CS can be paired with another stimulus to produce a further CR. The original CS serves as a UCS for the new association. **[S. p. 74]**

72 **Answer: D.** Lilliputian hallucinations are described as being pleasurable, and are associated with alcohol withdrawal. Autoscopic hallucinations are visual hallucinations of oneself, i.e. the phantom mirror image. Extracampine hallucinations are perceived outside one's field of perception. Hypnagogic hallucinations occur while going to sleep. **[D. pp. 30–1]**

73 A 50-year-old divorced unemployed man is brought into A&E from the police station by ambulance. He spent the last night in custody after the police caught him driving while intoxicated. According to the collateral from a police officer, this man became 'very mad' in the last few hours. He is least likely to present with:

A. Acute tremulousness.
B. Convulsions.
C. Sleep disturbance.
D. Staggering gait.
E. Transient hallucinosis.

74 Select the most correct statement regarding the *primacy effect* when individuals are forming impressions of people:

A. A positive first impression is more resistant to change than a negative one.
B. It is less powerful than the recency effect.
C. It is more important in forming impressions of strangers than friends.
D. It refers to the most important traits of an individual being identified.
E. It suggests information learned later about a person is more powerful.

75 Which one of the following terms is associated with Piaget's sensori-motor period of cognitive development?

A. Animism.
B. Compensation.
C. Conservation.
D. Object permanence.
E. Reversibility.

76 A researcher wishes to evaluate the attitudes of the general public to people with mental health problems. He designs a questionnaire using a Likert scale. What is the most likely source of bias associated with the use of this questionnaire?

A. Bias to middle.
B. Defensiveness.
C. Halo effect.
D. Hawthorn effect.
E. Response set.

73 **Answer: D.** Staggering gait is not a common feature of the alcohol withdrawal syndrome. It is one of the features in Wernicke's encephalopathy. The vignette in this question indicates an alcohol withdrawal presentation, which can commonly cause acute tremulousness, transient hallucinosis, convulsions and sleep disturbances. **[H. p. 124]**

74 **Answer: C.** The *primacy effect* (where there is a greater effect of what we learn first about a person) is contrasted with the *recency effect* (where there is a greater impact of information learned more recently). Generally, the primacy effect is the more powerful. A negative first impression is more resistant to change than is a positive first impression. It appears that the recency effect may be more important to people when forming opinions about family/friends while the primacy effect is more important for forming opinions of strangers. **[O. pp. 331–2]**

75 **Answer D.** Compensation, conservation, animism and reversibility are terms associated with the Concrete Operations stage of development. Object permanence is associated with the sensori-motor stage and refers to the child being aware of an object even when it is not in view. **[O. pp. 492–4]**

76 **Answer: A.** Responders on Likert scales are more likely to show a bias to the middle or the avoidance of extreme responses. Responders to a questionnaire on mental illness might also demonstrate the halo effect, allowing preconceptions to influence their responses. However, this is not the result of the Likert scale design of the questionnaire. **[S. p. 92]**

77 One of the features of 'secondary process' thinking described by Freud is listed below; other features relate to primary process. Which one is a feature of secondary process thinking?

A. Contradictions not recognised.

B. High tolerance of inconsistency.

C. Logical connections disregarded.

D. Reality principle.

E. Timelessness.

78 A 22-year-old man is admitted involuntarily for a relapse of his schizophrenic illness following non-concordance. The patient had poor insight and was adamant he did not want to be admitted. The clinicians believed the patient was at risk of further serious deterioration if he were not admitted. A mental health tribunal subsequently upheld the decision to detain the patient. Which (if any) of the duties imposed by the 'four principles' of bioethical practice has been breached by this action?

A. Beneficence.

B. Beneficence and justice.

C. Beneficence and respect for autonomy.

D. None of duties the four principles impose has been breached.

E. Nonmaleficence.

79 Jane is a 20-year-old woman with personality disorder and a history of multiple attempts of deliberate self-harm. Her mother is worried about the risk of completed suicide and has read something on the Internet about possible biochemical changes that are associated with completed suicide. From the list below, select the most appropriate evidence-based chemical change associated with suicide:

A. Decreased serotonin levels in the blood.

B. Decreased serotonin levels in CSF.

C. Lower 5-HIAA levels in CSF.

D. Lower VMA levels in urine.

E. Lower glutamate activity in brain.

80 A person who is at the conventional stage of Kohlberg's Morality Model obeys rules because he or she:

A. Believes in public welfare.   B. Believes in the principles of ethics.

C. Wants to avoid disapproval.   D. Wants to avoid punishment.

E. Wants to be rewarded.

77 **Answer: D.** Secondary process thinking is governed by the reality principle; primary process by the pleasure principle. Another feature of primary process thinking is lack of organisation. **[G. pp. 94–7]**

78 **Answer: E.** This answer, as with much in ethics, is debateable. Beneficence (doing good) has probably been achieved by admitting the patient to treat his illness. Justice has also been done by acting in accordance with the law and ensuring the patient gets appropriate treatment. Harm, however, has been done by doing something the patient does not want (being admitted and receiving treatment), therefore nonmaleficence has been breached. It can be debated whether the patient's autonomy is being respected: on the surface involuntary admission goes against this but one could argue that treatment restores autonomy in the incompetent patient. **[AM. pp. 33–9]**

79 **Answer: C.** Lower 5-HIAA levels in CSF are more strongly associated with completed suicide than with suicide attempts. 5-HIAA is a breakdown product of serotonin. **[H. p. 152]**

80 **Answer: C.** Obeying or ignoring rules because of a sense of ethics or society's good is associated with the post-conventional level. Obeying rules because of rewards or punishments is associated with the preconventional level, and obeying rules because of fear of disapproval or to be respected is associated with the conventional level. **[R. pp. 72–3]**

81 A 65-year-old man is referred for assessment by the cardiology team. He has a history of unstable angina and has become depressed. Which of the following antidepressants would be the most suitable for treating this man's depression?

A. Clomipramine.   B. Mirtazapine.

C. Phenelzine.   D. Reboxetine.

E. Venlafaxine.

82 A 19-year-old female patient, who lives with her parents and younger sister, attends your referral clinic for assessment. She describes a strained relationship with her mother and not being able to talk to her mother about their relationship. She admits that she is aggressive and verbally abusive to her younger sister over minor incidents. Which Freudian defence mechanism is she utilising?

A. Displacement.   B. Idealisation.

C. Identification.   D. Incorporation.

E. Splitting.

83 A 20-year-old single, unemployed man presented to A&E with euphoria, excitement, paranoid psychosis and tremor. On physical examination, he was tachycardic with slightly elevated blood pressure. He had a low-grade fever and both eyes showed mydriasis. You noted that his nasal septum was perforated. Abuse of which of the following would best explain this presentation?

A. Amphetamine.   B. Cocaine.

C. Crack cocaine.   D. Heroin.

E. LSD.

84 A 25-year-old man is taking part in a psychological experiment. He sits in a cubicle and sees a woman through the one-way glass at the front of the cubicle. There are five other one-way mirrors surrounding the woman in the centre: the man is told there are five other participants behind these, also taking part in the study. The woman (a stooge) suddenly clutches at her chest and falls to the floor, calling for help. What is the most likely response of the man?

A. He will do nothing.

B. He will look for help after a while.

C. He will look for help immediately.

D. He will start to cry.

E. He will try to break the one-way mirror.

81 **Answer: B.** Tricyclics and venlafaxine are the highest risk in treating patients with cardiac disease. MAOIs and reboxetine pose a moderate risk. Mirtazapine along with the SSRIs are believed to pose the lowest risk in patients with cardiac problems. **[X. p. 207]**

82 **Answer: A.** Displacement is the defence mechanism used by this patient. It is where emotions, ideas or wishes are transferred from their original object to a more acceptable substitute, in this case from the mother to her younger sister. Identification is where attributes of others are taken into oneself. Incorporation is where another's characteristics are taken on. Splitting involves dividing good objects, affects and memories from bad ones and is commonly used by patients with borderline personality disorder. **[G. pp. 103–4]**

83 **Answer: B.** Cocaine, which is most likely consumed by sniffing, produces euphoria, excitement, confusion, paranoid psychosis and formication. Its physical effects include: mydriasis, tremor, tachycardia, perforated nasal septum and fever. Heroin is likely to be abused intravenously while crack cocaine is by smoking. Amphetamines are likely to be taken either orally or intravenously and LSD is taken orally. **[H. pp. 138–9]**

84 **Answer: B.** This is an experiment looking at bystander intervention and in particular at the phenomenon of *diffusion of responsibility*. A similar experiment showed that all subjects looked for help if they thought they were the only one to witness someone in trouble. However, if they thought there other onlookers this response was reduced and delayed. While some did nothing, most looked for help but their response time was delayed in comparison to subjects who thought they were the sole witness. **[C. pp. 247–8]**

85 Componential and contextual sub-theories are associated with which theory of intelligence?

A. Burt and Vernon's hierarchical model.

B. Gardner's theory of multiple intelligences.

C. Spearman's two-factor theory.

D. Sternberg's triarchic theory.

E. Thurstone's primary mental abilities.

86 A 44-year-old man is attending for treatment of bipolar affective disorder. A routine blood investigation reveals a raised alkaline phosphatase (ALP) and gamma-glutamyl transpeptidase (GGT). Which of the following drugs is most likely to have caused this abnormality?

A. Carbamazepine.

B. Haloperidol.

C. Lithium.

D. Olanzapine.

E. Sodium valproate.

87 A seven-year-old boy was referred to your child psychiatry clinic. His parents described him as being defiant, disobedient and provocative in his behaviour, but say he has not carried out any acts that violate the law. Using ICD-10 criteria, which of the following diagnoses is the best fit for this boy?

A. Attention deficit/hyperkinetic disorder.

B. Conduct disorder.

C. Depressive conduct disorder.

D. Oppositional defiant disorder.

E. Social anxiety disorder.

88 Select one correct statement regarding Cattell's Sixteen Personality Factor (16PF) Test:

A. All 16 factors measure very different aspects of personality.

B. It is solely a self-report questionnaire.

C. It is used mainly in diagnosing an organic basis for personality change.

D. *Sober versus happy-go-lucky* is a factor.

E. There are objective tests involved which improve reliability.

85 **Answer: D.** Sternberg proposed the triarchic model which helps to explain, in an integrative way, the relationship between intelligence and the internal world (componential sub-theory), external world (contextual sub-theory) and the experience of the individual (experiential sub-theory). **[O. pp. 590–5]**

86 **Answer: A.** A raised ALP and GGT are potentially a sign of a hypersensitivity reaction to carbamazepine. Sodium valproate may very rarely cause fulminant hepatic failure, although all cases to date have occurred in children, often receiving multiple anticonvulsants with family histories of hepatic problems. **[V. p. 154]**

87 **Answer: D.** Oppositional defiant disorder is characterised by defiant, disobedient and provocative behaviour. The child should not have carried out any acts that violate the law. However, if more severe dissocial or aggressive acts are carried out, a conduct disorder diagnosis should be made. As there were no mood symptoms mentioned in the question, one cannot make a diagnosis of mixed disorders of conduct and emotions such as depressive conduct disorder. Attention deficit/hyperkinetic disorder and social anxiety disorders are distracters. **[I. pp. 268–73]**

88 **Answer: D.** A criticism of the 16PF has been that there is considerable overlap between the factors and so less than 16 personality traits are measured. There are different components to the test: Life (L) data (observer's ratings), Questionnaire (Q) data (self-report) and Objective test (T) data (assessment under controlled conditions). The T data have been found to be unreliable with different results being obtained on re-test conditions. It has not been described as a useful tool for organic personality change. **[C. pp. 331–3]**

89 You are collecting data on Class A drugs in order to start a research project. From the list below which is a Class A drug?

A. Amphetamines.

B. Barbiturates.

C. Benzodiazepines.

D. Cannabis.

E. LSD.

90 The Wechsler Adult Intelligence Score test comprises 11 sub-tests in two domains. Which one of the following is not a test in the Procedural domain?

A. Block design.

B. Digit span.

C. Object assembly.

D. Picture arrangement.

E. Picture completion.

91 A 50-year-old woman is attending for treatment of bipolar affective disorder. She has been on lithium for 10 years. Which of the following blood profiles is most likely in this woman?

A. $Ca^{2+}\uparrow$ Phosphate$\downarrow$.

B. $Ca^{2+}\downarrow$ Phosphate$\uparrow$.

C. T4$\downarrow$ T3$\uparrow$ TSH$\downarrow$.

D. T4$\uparrow$ T3$\downarrow$ TSH$\downarrow$.

E. T4$\uparrow$ T3$\uparrow$ TSH$\uparrow$.

92 A 65-year-old woman is referred by her GP with a history of short-term memory problems, and lack of spontaneity. Which one of the following tests is appropriate to test her frontal lobe function?

A. Dysgraphaesthesia.

B. Finger agnosia.

C. Interlocking finger test.

D. Interpretation of proverbs.

E. Rey's complex figure test.

89 **Answer: E.** Class A drugs are most of the opiates, cocaine, hallucinogens and psychotomimetics such as LSD, mescaline and PCP. Class B drugs are cannabis, codeine, amphetamines and barbiturates. Injectable forms of Class B drugs are designated as Class A. Class C drugs include dextropropoxyphene and the benzodiazepines. **[G. p. 236]**

90 **Answer: B.** Digit symbol is a Procedural sub-test whereas digit span is in the Verbal domain. **[R. p. 91]**

91 **Answer: A.** A raised Ca^{2+} and a lowered phosphate is characteristic of hyperparathyroidism which can be caused by long-term lithium therapy. Hypothyroidism, also caused by long-term lithium therapy, would be characterised by a lowered T4, a lowered T3 and a raised TSH. This thyroid profile is not represented in the options. **[X. pp. 379–82]**

92 **Answer: D.** Frontal lobe lesions can be tested for by digit span, Luria's verbal fluency test, cognitive estimates, serial 7s, and rhythm tapping tests. Interlocking finger test is a parietal lobe test; dysgraphaesthesia and finger agnosia are used to test parietal lobe function. The Rey complex figure is a visual test for occipital lobe function. See the *trickcyclists* website for revision of this topic. **[www.trickcyclists.co.uk/OSCEs]**

93 Which of the following psycho-social factors are least likely to be considered in the aetiology of alcohol dependence?

A. Modelling.

B. Occupation-related factors.

C. Operant conditioning.

D. Peer-group pressure.

E. The alcoholic personality.

94 Ali, a healthy five-year-old-boy of normal intelligence, takes part in a game with his mother and his cousin, Borat. Borat puts a ball into a box and then goes out to the garden for a few minutes. Ali's mother takes the ball out of the box and hides it in a drawer. She then asks Ali where he thinks Borat will look for the ball. What will Ali probably say?

A. 'Borat will forget.'

B. 'I don't know.'

C. 'In the box.'

D. 'In the drawer.'

E. 'In the garden.'

95 A child has depth perception, can accommodate fully, can link together two words and has full object permanence. What is the most likely minimum age of the child?

A. 2 months.

B. 6 months.

C. 12 months.

D. 18 months.

E. 36 months.

96 A 30-year-old man with diabetes mellitus is referred by his GP for treatment of depression. Which of the following antidepressants would be the most suitable?

A. Clomipramine.

B. Fluoxetine.

C. Mirtazapine.

D. Phenelzine.

E. Sertraline.

93 **Answer: E.** There is little evidence of an 'alcoholic personality'. Modelling may explain familial association. Operant conditioning may be seen whereby relief of withdrawal symptoms promotes further abuse. The role of alcohol in social activities has been considered as well as cultural values. Peer-group pressure and occupation-related factors have also been considered as important. **[H. p. 123]**

94 **Answer: C.** Simon Baron-Cohen conducted a study in 1985 to test the theory of mind hypothesis among normal children, children with Down's syndrome and children with autism. Most of the normal children (age range three to five) passed the test. The theory of mind refers to the child being able to distinguish between what he knows as opposed to what someone else would know. Irrelevantly, Prof. Baron-Cohen is the cousin of Sacha Baron Cohen (of Ali G and *Borat* fame). **[O. pp. 580–1]**

95 **Answer: D.** Children develop object permanence between 12 and 18 months of age. Depth perception is present by 6 months and accommodation is also fully developed at 6 months. Children can link two words together between 18 and 24 months **[O. pp. 237, 281, 492]**

96 **Answer: E.** The antidepressant of choice in a patient with diabetes is sertraline. Fluoxetine can cause hypoglycaemia, and its side-effects (tremor, sweating, nausea, anxiety) may be mistaken for hypoglycaemia. MAOIs may reduce serum glucose by up to 30% by their direct influence on the pathway of gluconeogenesis. Tricyclics may adversely affect diabetic control as they increase serum glucose levels by up to 150%, increase carbohydrate craving and reduce the metabolic rate. The manufacturers of mirtazapine recommend care, although there are no reports of problems. **[X. pp. 215–17]**

97 A newborn baby possesses which of the following visual characteristics?

A. Depth perception.

B. Fixed focus.

C. Object completion.

D. Perceptual constancy.

E. Colour vision.

98 With regard to the Wechsler Adult Intelligence Scale (WAIS-R), choose the correct statement from the following:

A. A sophisticated theory of intelligence underlies the test.

B. All sub-tests are timed.

C. Digit span is included on the performance scale.

D. It is the most commonly used IQ test in the world.

E. The verbal and performance scales comprise six sub-tests each.

99 Albert has started smoking since he saw a famous football star smoking on television. This behaviour can be best explained by which of the following?

A. Imprinting.

B. Latent learning.

C. Positive reinforcement.

D. Pro-social behaviour.

E. Social learning theory.

100 Which of the following Gestalt laws best explains how many musical notes make a melody?

A. Continuity.

B. *Gestalten*.

C. Minimum principle.

D. Proximity.

E. Similarity.

97 **Answer: B.** Fixed focus is present at birth. Depth perception, object completion, perceptual constancy, and colour vision are acquired abilities. **[F. pp. 6–7]**

98 **Answer: D.** The WAIS-R is atheoretical and comprises two scales: the verbal scale (which includes digit span) has six sub-tests which are not timed while the performance scale which has five sub-tests which are timed. It is the most commonly used IQ test in the world. **[O. p. 598]**

99 **Answer: E.** Research suggests that much of our behaviour is in reference to other people and is acquired through observational learning. Prosocial behaviour is a positive behaviour and the opposite of antisocial behaviour. Latent learning is a type of learning in which learned material is not expressed until considerably later. **[AC. p. 79]**

100 **Answer: D.** Continuity explains how speech is perceived, proximity explains how elements appearing near each other tend to be perceived together (an auditory example would be the perception of a series of musical notes as a melody). Similarity explains how voices combine in a choir. The minimum principle states that we will perceive stimuli in the simplest way. *Gestalten* simply means 'patterns'. **[O. p. 211]**

101 A 22-year-old woman is referred by her GP who reports that she has anorexia nervosa. Following your assessment you are of the opinion that this woman has bulimia nervosa. Which of the following features in her history would most support your diagnosis?

A. Bingeing episodes.

B. Body Mass Index of 22.5.

C. Morbid fear of fatness.

D. Persistent preoccupation with eating.

E. Self-induced vomiting.

102 According to object relations theory, personality is shaped by early parental relationships. Which of the following traits would result from struggle with parents for control?

A. Antisocial traits.   B. Borderline traits.

C. Dependent traits.   D. Hysterical traits.

E. Obsessive compulsive traits.

103 Which one of the following is not relevant to the understanding of the genetics of personality disorders?

A. Concordance rates for psychopathy in MZ twins are higher than in DZ twins.

B. Danish adoption studies.

C. Female criminals have higher genetic loading than males.

D. Relatives of females with Briquet's syndrome have high rates of antisocial personality disorder.

E. Swedish army conscript study.

104 Psychiatric anthropology suggests the following adult psychiatric syndromes can be found cross-culturally, except:

A. Bipolar disorder.   B. Brief reactive psychoses.

C. Bulimia nervosa.   D. Major depression.

E. Schizophrenia.

101 **Answer: B.** Bulimia nervosa and anorexia nervosa share a number of features, including a morbid fear of fatness, a preoccupation with eating, vomiting or purging behaviour, and binge eating. The diagnosis of anorexia requires a BMI of <17.5, and amenorrhea. However, it should be remembered that 15% of patients with anorexia progress to bulimia. **[H. pp. 93–100]**

102 **Answer: E.** Dependent personality traits are thought to result from maternal deprivation. Obsessive compulsive traits come from struggles with parents for control. Hysterical traits come from parental seduction and competition and borderline traits from a lack of stable attachment during development. **[G. p. 346]**

103 **Answer: E.** The Swedish army conscript study investigated the relationship between cannabis use and the development of psychosis. All the other statements are relevant. **[H. p. 86]**

104 **Answer: C.** Apart from certain anxiety disorders and A, B, D, E listed in the question, most of the DSM-IV listed diagnoses are found mainly in the US and Europe and thus could be said to be culture-bound. **[M. p. 302]**

105 In operant conditioning which of the following reinforcement schedules is the most resistant to extinction of the response?

A. Continuous reinforcement. B. Fixed interval.

C. Fixed ratio. D. Variable interval.

E. Variable ratio.

106 A 35-year-old married man, who is long-term unemployed, is referred for assessment to the outpatient department. He is accompanied by his concerned wife. He reports to you that he was seriously assaulted three months previously. He was attacked by two men, who drove him around in the boot of a car for two hours, before holding a gun to his head and threatening to shoot him. He was then beaten and left on the side of the road. He has a post-traumatic stress disorder. He also has a history of depression. Which of the following features in this man's case would improve this man's prognosis?

A. Duration of the trauma. B. Pre-morbid function.

C. Psychiatric history. D. Severity of the trauma.

E. Social support.

107 Using ICD-10 criteria which one of the features below is common to anorexia and bulimia nervosa?

A. Amenorrhoea.

B. Attempts to counteract the fattening effects of food.

C. Morbid fear of fatness.

D. Persistent preoccupation with eating.

E. Self-induced weight loss.

108 In overcoming barriers to communication with the patient, which of the following is most important for the doctor?

A. Being empathic. B. Being hard-working.

C. Being self-sacrificing. D. Liking to help.

E. Liking to solve problems.

105 **Answer: E.** The order is: Variable Ratio>Variable Interval>Fixed Interval = Fixed ratio>Continuous reinforcement. **[O. p. 152]**

106 **Answer: E.** Good prognostic factors in post-traumatic stress disorder are a healthy pre-morbid function, a brief trauma of lesser severity, no personal history of psychiatric illness, and good social support. In this man's case he has a number of poor prognostic factors. However, he appears to have the support of his partner. **[H. p. 74]**

107 **Answer: C.** The specific psychopathology of a morbid fear of fatness is common to both. **[I. pp. 176–9]**

108 **Answer: A.** Empathy is crucial and is defined in the quoted text as 'the ability to reflect accurately the inner experience of another person'. While each of the other traits can of course be helpful in some circumstances, in excess they can hinder the consultation, as can traits such as arrogance and risk aversion. **[M. pp. 87–8]**

109 Sharon believes that David Beckham (the football star) is in love with her even though she has never met him and has never contacted him. She retains this belief despite being ridiculed by her family and friends. Which of the following best suits her presentation?

A. Capgras' syndrome.   B. De Clerambault's syndrome.

C. Ekbom's syndrome.   D. Fregoli syndrome.

E. Othello syndrome.

110 Tolman and Honzik's theory which explains how animals learn without reinforcement is known as?

A. Classical conditioning.   B. Insight learning.

C. Latent learning.   D. Operant learning.

E. Premack's principle.

111 You have been seeing a 45-year-old man who presented with symptoms of depression and post-traumatic symptoms following an accident at work. He has shown little response to antidepressant medication at high doses and the diagnosis remains unclear. You refer him for psychological assessment. Which of the following instruments would you expect the psychologist to use?

A. Adaptive Behaviour Scales.

B. Brief Psychiatric Rating Scale.

C. CAGE.

D. General Health Questionnaire.

E. Minnesota Multiphasic Personality Inventory.

112 A 31-year-old man with a fear of flying is advised by a friend to go on a long-haul flight to help him overcome his fear. Which one of the terms below best describes this advice?

A. Cognitive analytic therapy.   B. Flooding.

C. Implosive therapy.   D. Solution focused therapy.

E. Systematic desensitisation.

109 **Answer: B.** Erotomania is considered a delusion of being loved, generally by someone of superior social status, and is more common in females. Ekbom's syndrome has also been called delusional parasitosis. Othello syndrome is characterised by delusions of jealousy and infidelity. Capgras' syndrome and Fregoli syndrome are both delusions of misidentification. **[D. pp. 117–18]**

110 **Answer: C.** Pavlov is associated with classical conditioning. Latent learning was postulated by Tolman and Honzik following experiments in which rats seemed to learn their way around a maze without a reward to reinforce the behaviour. Reinforcement is associated with operant conditioning. Premack's principle states that any high-frequency behaviour can be used as a reinforcer. Insight learning is a purely cognitive theory that stems from the Gestalt movement. **[O. p. 155]**

111 **Answer: E.** The Minnesota Multiphasic Personality Inventory (MMPI) is a self-rated questionnaire validated on psychiatric patients and is used to identify psychopathology and one's personality profile. The Adaptive Behaviour Scales are used in patients with intellectual disability. The Brief Psychiatric Rating Scale is used to measure psychotic symptoms and psychopathology. The CAGE is a brief screening tool for alcohol abuse. The General Health Questionnaire is a commonly used screening tool used in primary care and general population studies. **[H. pp. 6–8]**

112 **Answer: B.** Flooding is being described here, i.e. exposure of a patient to a phobic object in a non-graded manner with no attempts to reduce anxiety beforehand. If flooding is conducted using the imagination, it is referred to as implosive therapy. Systematic desensitisation involves relaxation training prior to graded exposure of phobic items. Items A and D are distracters. **[A. pp. 852–3]**

113 A 61-year-old single unemployed man is admitted to the psychiatric ward with alcohol dependence syndrome and is in an advanced withdrawal state. Which of the following management lines is least likely to be effective?

A. Anticonvulsant administration.

B. Attention to general medical condition.

C. Benzodiazepine administration.

D. Hydration should be encouraged.

E. Thiamine administration.

114 In interviewing the family, which of the following is recommended?

A. Allowing just the family members who have strong views to speak.

B. Becoming particularly close with helpful family members.

C. Getting each family member to comment on the problem.

D. Promising each member that you will keep secrets.

E. Taking sides with the family members who are in the right.

115 The concept present in the pre-operational stage whereby a child may remark that 'the sun went because Daddy took it away' is called what?

A. Animism.

B. Artificialism.

C. Centration.

D. Creationism.

E. Hypothetical deductive reasoning.

116 A 22-year-old patient presents with a movement disorder. He demonstrates rapid sudden blinking. This movement is more noticeable when the patient is anxious. His partner reports that does not occur when he is asleep, and that it is less prominent when he is concentrating on an activity. What type of movement is this patient displaying?

A. Dyskinesia.

B. Hemiballismic movements.

C. Myoclonic movements.

D. Tics.

E. Torticollis.

113 **Answer: A.** Anticonvulsants may have a limited role for some patients such as a planned detoxification in a patient with a history of seizures. However, this would have to be commenced before the detox: in this vignette, anticonvulsants are likely to be of little benefit because of the time required for them to become effective. **[M. pp. 495–6]**

114 **Answer: C.** It is important to allow all family members an opportunity to give their views on the problem. Taking sides is likely to lead to resentment among some family members, thereby hindering the process. The clinician has to respect confidentiality of course but should not make sweeping promises about keeping secrets. **[M. p. 91]**

115 **Answer: B.** Artificialism occurs when the child believes that events in the world are caused by people's actions. **[R. p. 71]**

116 **Answer: D.** Tics are rapid purposeless movements of a functionally related group of muscles. They are most commonly facial. They increase with anxiety and decrease during sleep. They may be reduced during periods of sustained attention. Myoclonic movements may be distinguished from tics as they affect a whole muscle or part of a muscle but not muscle groups. Dystonic movements are slower and more sustained than tics. Hemiballismic movements are movements of the limbs, which are coarse, intermittent and unilateral. Dyskinetic movements which tend to occur in the facial muscles, e.g. tardive dyskinesia, also affect muscle groups but are slower than tics. Torticollis involves the gradual development of tonic spasms in the neck muscles. **[H. p. 285]**

117 The psychiatric symptom of multiple sclerosis (MS) that occurs most commonly during the early course of the illness is?

A. Depression.

B. Euphoria.

C. Hypomania.

D. Hysteria.

E. Psychosis.

118 Pre-morbid IQ in a man with brain injury to the frontal lobes may be estimated from all of the following except:

A. Educational record.

B. Estimation ability.

C. Occupational record.

D. Reading ability.

E. Vocabulary.

119 In a long-stay ward a patient with chronic schizophrenia has a tendency to stay in an immobile position for a long time. This condition is best described by which of the following terms?

A. Akinesia.

B. Catalepsy.

C. Cataplexy.

D. Catatonic rigidity.

E. Obtundation.

120 Which one of the following adult attachment styles is not associated with the Adult Attachment Interview (AAI)?

A. Autonomous.

B. Dismissing.

C. Disorganised.

D. Preoccupied.

E. Unresolved.

117 **Answer: A.** Traditionally, it was thought that euphoria was the commonest mood disorder seen in MS. However, depression is seen just as commonly, and usually earlier in the illness, particularly after diagnosis, with euphoria occurring later in the course. Hypomania has been reported with steroid use. Presentation with psychosis is rare, and hysteria has also been reported. **[L. pp. 694–8]**

118 **Answer: B.** Reading and vocabulary are associated with IQ and are 'overlearned' so may be of use in estimating the brain-injured patient's pre-morbid IQ. The patient's education and occupational records are crude but still of use in this regard. Estimation is dependent on frontal lobe functioning and thus may be severely affected in this situation. **[M. pp. 98–9]**

119 **Answer: B.** Catalepsy is a general term for an immobile position that is constantly maintained. Cataplexy is a temporary loss of muscle tone and weakness precipitated by a variety of emotional states. Catatonic rigidity is a voluntary assumption of rigid posture that is held against all efforts to be moved while akinesia is a lack of physical movement. Obtundation refers to decreased alertness and slowed responses. **[K. p. 281]**

120 **Answer: C.** *Disorganised* is an attachment style described by Ainsworth. The other attachment types are adult attachment types described by Main (AAI). **[T. p. 58]**

121 A 35-year-old married woman with a history of depression presents in the outpatient department complaining of loss of libido. Which antidepressant would be the most suitable to prescribe to address this side-effect?

A. Fluoxetine.

B. Lofepramine.

C. Phenelzine.

D. Mirtazapine.

E. Venlafaxine.

122 A 25-year-old male pedestrian is hit by a car crossing the road; he suffers a head injury as a result. On neurological examination, it is noted that his right pupil is dilated. Which of the following causes is the most likely to give this clinical picture?

A. Brain death.

B. Brainstem injury.

C. Narcotic overdose.

D. Pontine injury.

E. Subarachnoid haemorrhage.

123 Which of the following is not relevant in relation to providing informed consent?

A. Competency.

B. Decision.

C. Disclosure of information.

D. Tarasoff doctrine.

E. Voluntariness.

124 The ecological validity of neuropsychological test results may be improved by:

A. Increased reliance on test data.

B. Short test sessions.

C. Stressing the importance of the test to the patient.

D. Test anxiety.

E. Using tests that reflect real-life tasks.

121 **Answer: D.** Mirtazapine has a lower incidence of sexual side-effects than most other antidepressants at 24%. SSRIs may indirectly decrease libido through a direct inhibition of sexual arousal and orgasm. Tricyclic anti-depressants may decrease libido indirectly through sedation. Venlafaxine can inhibit arousal and orgasm. **[X. pp. 195–7]**

122 **Answer: E.** Subarachnoid haemorrhage, subdural haematoma, and raised intracranial pressure can give this sign, i.e. one dilated pupil. Pontine haemorrhage and narcotic overdose are suggested by very small pupils. **[AO. p. 393]**

123 **Answer: D.** The Tarasoff doctrine refers to a court decision that a therapist who discovers risk towards a third party must take all reasonable steps to protect this person. Informed consent, verbal or written, involves disclosure of information, competency, understanding, voluntariness and decision making and recording. **[www.gmc-uk.org/ guidance/ethical_guidance/consent_guidance/Consent_guidance. pdf]**

124 **Answer: E.** The ecological validity of a test refers to how well a test result will predict functioning on a real-life task. Being focused just on the result numbers the test throws up may miss background information on how the patient may perform in real life. Short test sessions may miss the effects of fatigue which is when real-life problems are often seen. Test anxiety may inhibit the patient whereas priming the patient regarding the importance of the test may throw up unrepresentative results. **[M. pp. 100–1]**

125 The correct order of stages of Kübler-Ross's anticipatory grief is?

A. Acceptance, Anger, Denial, Bargaining, Depression.

B. Anger, Denial, Bargaining, Disorganisation, Acceptance.

C. Denial, Anger, Bargaining, Depression, Acceptance.

D. Shock, Anger, Guilt, Denial, Depression.

E. Numbness, Yearning, Disorganisation, Reorganisation.

126 A 25-year-old woman with a diagnosis of schizophrenia presents to the outpatient department. She reports that she is being sexually assaulted every night by terrorists. Which of the following perceptual abnormalities is she most likely to be experiencing?

A. Autoscopic hallucinations.

B. Haptic hallucinations.

C. Hygric hallucinations.

D. Hypnagogic hallucinations.

E. Kinaesthetic hallucinations.

127 Which of the cranial nerves is not routinely tested when performing a neurological examination?

A. Abducens nerve.

B. Oculomotor nerve.

C. Olfactory nerve.

D. Trigeminal nerve.

E. Trochlear nerve.

128 A 27-year-old man claims to have various cognitive difficulties following a fight in which his head was injured. The man is due to be prosecuted for having started the fight and there has been the suggestion he is malingering to avoid his legal difficulties. Which of the following from neuropsychological tests would *least* support malingering?

A. He finds easy tests as hard as difficult ones.

B. His recognition recall is better than his free recall.

C. He responds to tests with marked slowness but converses normally.

D. On true-or-false questions he gets all questions wrong.

E. Over time his test results worsen.

125 **Answer: C.** Kübler-Ross interviewed over 200 terminally ill people and found common stages of grief. However, they are probably culturally specific, but have led to other theories. **[T. p. 61]**

126 **Answer: B.** Haptic hallucinations are superficial hallucinations of touch. The hallucination may be delusionally elaborated. Hygric hallucinations are superficial hallucinations of fluid. Kinaesthetic hallucinations are those of muscle or joint sense. Hypnagogic hallucinations are perceptions which occur while going asleep. Autoscopic hallucinations are abnormalities of visual perceptions involving seeing oneself. **[D. pp. 89–90]**

127 **Answer: C.** The olfactory nerve is not routinely tested. If the patient complains of anosmia, it is tested using bottles with smells such as vanilla, peppermint and coffee. Pungent smells should be avoided when testing for olfactory nerve function, as noxious stimuli are carried by sensory fibres of the fifth cranial nerve. **[AO. p. 320]**

128 **Answer: B.** Malingering may be suspected when a pattern emerges from various test results or from the patient's behaviour regarding the tests. Patients with genuine head injuries tend to have consistent test performance with behaviour out of test situations, perform better on easier tests than hard ones and show some improvement on tests over time. Getting all true-or-false questions wrong suggests knowing the answers and selecting the wrong answer deliberately. Patients even with genuine head injuries tend to do better on recognition recall than free recall (having no prompts). **[M. p. 100]**

129 John wants to marry Julia who suffers from schizophrenia. There is no history of schizophrenia for John or his family. They plan to have one child. They attend your clinic for counselling regarding the chance their child might develop schizophrenia. What will be your answer?

A. 1%.

B. 6%.

C. 13%.

D. 20%.

E. 40%.

130 Which of the following is not a trait associated with Minuchin's 'psycho-somatic family'?

A. Enmeshment.

B. Critical.

C. Lack of conflict resolution.

D. Overprotective.

E. Rigid.

131 A 26-year-old man is seen following a road traffic accident in which he sustained serious head and limb injuries. He is noted to have palsy in his left arm. Which of the following features would suggest that the upper limb paralysis results from an upper rather than a lower motor neuron lesion?

A. Babinski sign.

B. Fasciculation.

C. Flaccid paralysis.

D. Hyporeflexia.

E. Hypotonia.

132 Which one of the clinical features listed below occurs in bulbar palsy?

A. Absent gag reflex.

B. Increased jaw jerk.

C. Labile emotions.

D. Spastic tongue.

E. Spastic dysarthria.

129 **Answer: C.** If there is one parent affected, the risk of developing schizophrenia in the children is 12–15%. This is increased to 40% if both parents have schizophrenia. The highest risk is in identical twins, which is 46%. If one sibling has schizophrenia, the risk of developing schizophrenia is 12–15%. **[AB. p. 191]**

130 **Answer: B.** A 'critical' trait is not described by Minuchin as being a characteristic of the 'psychosomatic family'. Critical comments, however, can be a trait in families that can increase the risk of relapse of schizophrenia in one of its members. **[T. pp. 222, 260]**

131 **Answer: A.** An upper motor neuron lesion will be characterised by hypertonia, spastic paralysis, hyperreflexia and the Babinski sign. A lower motor neuron lesion will be characterised by hypotonia, flaccid paralysis, hyporeflexia and muscles wasting with fasciculation and fibrillation. **[S. p. 29]**

132 **Answer: A.** Signs B to E, along with increased or normal gag reflex, are indicative of a pseudobulbar palsy (bilateral upper motor neuron lesion of IX, X and XII cranial nerves). Bulbar palsy has absent gag, wasted or fasciculations of the tongue, absent or normal jaw jerk, nasal speech and normal emotions. **[AO. p. 345]**

133 Which of the following is least likely to be a long-term consequence of maternal deprivation?

A. Antisocial behaviour.

B. Depression.

C. Despair and detachment.

D. Developmental delay.

E. Poor growth.

134 Select the most correct statement about ICD-10:

A. ICD-10 distinguishes conversion from dissociation.

B. ICD-10 does not use the term 'neurotic'.

C. Passive-aggressive personality disorder is mentioned in ICD-10.

D. The diagnosis of schizophrenia requires symptoms for at least six months.

E. The term 'neurasthenia' is not used.

135 Peeking through the door in the psychotherapy unit you notice the co-therapist looking through a one-way mirror at a family undergoing therapy. What type of therapy are you witnessing?

A. Balint group therapy.

B. Milan school style.

C. Strategic family therapy.

D. Structural family therapy.

E. Systemic family therapy.

136 A 55-year-old man with a history of alcohol dependence syndrome is referred by the A&E registrar who reports that he has Wernicke's encephalopathy. Following your assessment you are of the opinion that he has progressed to Korsakoff's syndrome. Which of the following features would be most supportive of your diagnosis?

A. Confabulation.

B. Confusion/clouding of consciousness.

C. Nystagmus.

D. Peripheral neuropathy.

E. Staggering gait.

133 **Answer: C.** The distress syndrome is considered to be a consequence of short-term separation and it includes protest, despair and detachment. Consequences of long-term maternal deprivation include the other items in the question and also poor development of IQ and language and affectionless psychopathy. **[H. p. 293]**

134 **Answer: C.** Passive-aggressive and narcissistic personality disorders are mentioned in the inclusions under 'other specific personality disorders'. DSM-IV distinguishes conversion from dissociation; ICD-10 does not. The term 'neurotic' is retained mainly as a descriptive term: originally it was planned to omit the term altogether. DSM-IV requires six months of symptoms for schizophrenia whereas ICD-10 needs just one month. DSM-IV does not use the term 'neurasthenia' but ICD-10 does (F48.0). **[M. pp. 113–14]**

135 **Answer: D.** Structural family therapy is associated with Minuchin. He researched the links between social poverty and childhood psychological problems, and pioneered the use of the one-way mirror. Systemic theory is synonymous with the Milan group. Strategic family therapy perceives the fact of the complaint about a child as the problem rather than focusing on the problem itself. **[T. p. 557; W. p. 241]**

136 **Answer: A.** Korsakoff's syndrome is characterised by the inability to form new memories and retrograde amnesia, confabulation, relative preservation of other intellectual functions, clear consciousness and peripheral neuropathy. The presentation of Wernicke's encephalopathy also involves peripheral neuropathy, with ocular palsies and nystagmus, ataxia, confusion and clouding of consciousness. **[H. p. 125]**

137 Which of the following behaviours occurs when a couple have a child, and rear that child together?

A. Both parents display increased autonomy.

B. Both parents display less affection to each other.

C. Both parents display more feminine behaviours.

D. Power is shared across the generations within the family.

E. Rules are always explicit within the new family.

138 Select the most correct statement about schizophrenia (ICD-10):

A. Affective changes are rare in hebephrenic schizophrenia.

B. Delusions of bodily change are uncommon in paranoid schizophrenia.

C. Schizophrenic symptoms may be absent in post-schizophrenic depression.

D. Visual hallucinations are rarely predominant in paranoid schizophrenia.

E. Vivid hallucinations invalidate a diagnosis of catatonic schizophrenia.

139 The manager of your hospital wants to build a new day hospital and is interested to know about new cases of schizophrenia. Your city has a population of 100 000. How many new cases will you expect to develop over a period of one year?

A. 1.

B. 5.

C. 15.

D. 30.

E. 100.

140 Yalom described a number of group specific therapeutic factors. Which of the following is not one of them?

A. Altruism.

B. Cohesiveness.

C. Insight.

D. Interpersonal learning.

E. Tension.

137 **Answer: C.** Both parents exhibit more feminine behaviour, and their relationship becomes more affectionate, despite the possible stresses involved, i.e. sleep deprivation, reduced income etc. Rules are often but not always explicit and are understood by all family members. **[F. p. 57; AP. p. 269]**

138 **Answer: D.** Affective changes are common in hebephrenic schizophrenia. Common delusions in paranoid schizophrenia include delusions of persecution, jealousy and bodily change. The diagnosis of post-schizophrenic depression requires that some schizophrenic symptoms are present. Vivid hallucination may occur in catatonic schizophrenia as an oneiroid state. Paranoid schizophrenia is associated with visual hallucinations but it is rare for them to predominate. **[I. pp. 86–95]**

139 **Answer: C.** The incidence of schizophrenia in the UK and US is around 15 new cases per 100 000 per year. The lifetime risk of schizophrenia is 7–13 per 1000 population. The point prevalence is 2–5 per 1000. **[AB. p. 190]**

140 **Answer: E.** Common group tension was described by Ezriel. **[T. p. 558]**

141 A 36-year-old woman attends for assessment at the outpatient clinic. She reports that she has been previously diagnosed with 'seasonal affective disorder'. Which of the following features of her depression is not supportive of this diagnostic term?

A. Hyperphagia.

B. Insomnia.

C. Loss of interest.

D. Low energy.

E. Symptoms worsening in the months of November to February.

142 A nine-year-old boy who breaks a window in his parents' home with his football worries about the consequences when his parents find out. Using Kohlberg's theory, at what stage is the boy in his moral development?

A. Approval/disapproval.

B. Authority orientation.

C. Punishment.

D. Reward.

E. Social contract.

143 You are seeing a 21-year-old man for psychoanalytic psychotherapy. Over the last number of sessions you have noted that he is displaying warm feelings towards you. Which of the following describes your patient's attitude?

A. Counter-transference.

B. Displacement.

C. Reaction formation.

D. Therapeutic alliance.

E. Transference.

144 Which is the most correct statement regarding ICD-10 depressive episode?

A. Feelings of guilt are uncommon in mild episodes.

B. It may be diagnosed if symptoms are present for less than two weeks.

C. Predominance of anxiety as a symptom invalidates the diagnosis.

D. The somatic syndrome usually requires three somatic symptoms.

E. Weight loss is defined as 10% or more of body weight in the last month.

141 **Answer: B.** Seasonal affective disorder was a term used to describe patients who recognised a seasonal pattern to their mood and described consistent atypical symptoms of hypersomnia, hyperphagia, along with tiredness, and low mood in winter. Community studies have not supported the existence of a specific syndrome, although there is some seasonality in mood disorder. **[A. p. 407]**

142 **Answer: A.** He is at the approval/disapproval stage of his moral development. At this stage the emphasis is on having good intentions and on ways of behaving that conform to most people's views of good behaviour. **[F. p. 53; C. p. 177]**

143 **Answer: E.** Transference is important in the psychotherapeutic relationship: it may provide aetiological clues as well as an important therapeutical tool for interpretation. There is often an erotic component which may be difficult or impossible for the patient to admit. **[M. p. 1437]**

144 **Answer: B.** Symptoms usually need to be present for at least two weeks but the text suggests rapid onset of severe symptoms may allow an earlier diagnosis. Feelings of guilt are common even in mild episodes. Anxiety symptoms may dominate the clinical picture at times. The somatic syndrome usually needs four of the somatic symptoms (such as early morning waking or loss of libido). Weight loss is usually defined as loss of at least 5% of body weight in the last month. **[I. pp. 119–21]**

145 Which of the following statements concerning Carl Rogers is false?

A. He pioneered Client Centred Therapy.

B. He believed in the importance of genuineness, unconditional positive regard and empathic understanding as key attributes of therapists.

C. He developed the Q-sort technique.

D. He applied the nomothetic approach to personality.

E. He rejected all diagnostic labelling.

146 A 25-year-old man who has been attending the service for treatment of anxiety is involved in a road traffic accident. Which of the following factors increases this man's risk for significant cognitive sequelae?

A. Glasgow Coma Scale score of 13 following the accident.

B. No intracranial bleeding.

C. Non-penetrating injury.

D. Post-traumatic amnesia of five to six days.

E. Retrograde amnesia covering minutes before the accident.

147 A 31-year-old woman presents to you for psychiatric assessment. She believes that her new home has listening devices planted by her work colleagues. This belief began suddenly when she noticed the cables from her pre-installed house alarm. Her symptoms are best described by which of the following?

A. Delusional perception.

B. Made feeling.

C. Somatic delusion.

D. Somatic passivity.

E. Thought broadcast.

148 Select the most correct statement regarding ICD-10 eating disorders:

A. Bulimia nervosa is often associated with a history of an episode of anorexia nervosa.

B. In anorexia nervosa body weight is at least 20% below expected weight.

C. Pica is not included in ICD-10 eating disorders.

D. The diagnosis of anorexia nervosa is unreliable.

E. The presence of vaginal bleeding invalidates a diagnosis of anorexia nervosa.

145 **Answer: D.** Rogers believed in the idiographic approach which maintains that all humans are unique and therefore not measurable on common dimensions. Measuring such dimensions would be a nomothetic approach. **[O. p. 610, 676]**

146 **Answer: D.** A post-traumatic amnesia of two to seven days indicates severe injury and residual damage. A Glasgow Coma Score of 13–15 suggests mild injury. The shorter the period of retrograde amnesia the less severe the injury; this amnesia is not very useful for prognosis. A penetrating head injury and intracranial bleeding would worsen the prognosis but this man sustained neither. **[A. pp. 309–10, AW. pp. 170–1]**

147 **Answer: A.** Delusional perception is where a delusion arrives fully fledged on the basis of a real perception, which others would regard as commonplace and unrelated. **[A. p. 371; G. pp. 88–9]**

148 **Answer: A.** The interval between the anorexic episode and bulimic episode can vary from months to years. In anorexia the weight is at least 15% below that expected or the BMI is 17.5 or less. Pica of nonorganic origin in adults is included under *other eating disorders* (F50.8). The diagnosis of anorexia is reliable since the symptoms are easily recognised and clinicians tend to agree on diagnosis. While amenorrhoea is usually present in anorexia, vaginal bleeding may occur in women taking the oral contraceptive pill. **[I. pp. 176–81]**

149 James has recently been admitted to your ward with schizophrenia. While reading about his condition on the Internet, his mother has discovered that he may be at increased risk of suicide. She asks you what the risk of suicide in patients with schizophrenia is. What will you answer?

A. 1%.   B. 5%.

C. 15%.   D. 50%.

E. 80%.

150 Which one of the following would you do to protect against a multi-disciplinary team (a group) making polarised and therefore riskier decisions?

A. Appoint a 'devil's advocate'.

B. Appoint a directive leader.

C. Appoint a persuasive leader.

D. Appoint 'mindguards'.

E. Ensure high stress levels at the meeting.

151 A 36-year-old man who is being treated for depression complains that he has been experiencing sleep difficulties. He reports that his wife complains he appears frightened and shouts in his sleep at night. He has no recollection of the incidents on waking. What type of sleep disturbance is this man describing?

A. Narcolepsy.   B. Night terrors.

C. Nightmares.   D. Sleep drunkenness.

E. Somnambulism.

152 A 17-year-old girl who is otherwise healthy and has a normal weight is brought to a dentist by her parents for treatment of toothache. Her dentist notes dental erosion and parotid gland enlargement. Which psychiatric diagnosis is most likely in this case?

A. Anorexia nervosa.   B. Binge-eating disorder.

C. Bulimia nervosa.   D. Depressive disorder.

E. Paranoid schizophrenia.

149 **Answer: C.** Suicide is the most common cause of premature death in schizophrenia. It accounts for 10–38% of all deaths happening in schizophrenia. The highest risk period is in the first year after presentation. **[AB. p. 190]**

150 **Answer: A.** Answers B, C, D and E are all conducive to 'groupthink' and therefore to polarised and poorly thought-out decisions. Appointing a 'devil's advocate' will help the group to consider alternatives. **[T. p. 81]**

151 **Answer: B.** Night terrors occur in deep sleep early in the night. They more typically occur in childhood, but can occur in adulthood. The person displays intense anxiety, may shout, and has a rapid pulse and respiration. Usually there is complete amnesia for the experience on waking. This latter point distinguishes night terrors from nightmares, a type of dream, which is remembered vividly if the person awakes immediately after the experience. Narcolepsy is characterised by short episodes of sleep which occur irresistibly during the day. Somnambulism is another term for sleepwalking. Sleep drunkenness is the complaint of feeling drowsy, incompetent and uncoordinated for a prolonged period of time on waking. **[D. pp. 40–3]**

152 **Answer: C.** Bulimia nervosa is most likely as this 17 year old has a normal weight, and the dental problems suggest complications from repeated vomiting. Binge-eating disorder is not the diagnosis as repeated vomiting is not a feature of that condition. In schizophrenia dental problems should be considered due to poor self-care. **[I. pp. 176–81]**

153 Regarding suitability for dynamic psychotherapy, which of the following is not correct?

   A. Ability to form and sustain therapeutic relationships is required.

   B. Ability to understand problems in psychological terms is required.

   C. Adequate ego strength is required.

   D. Phobia is a contraindication.

   E. Psychosis is a contraindication.

154 Select the most correct statement regarding DSM-IV schizoaffective disorder:

   A. Depressive symptoms rarely meet criteria for a major depressive episode.

   B. Mood symptoms and psychotic symptoms alternate.

   C. Mood symptoms need to be present for at least two weeks.

   D. The minimum duration of a schizoaffective episode is one month.

   E. There are two subtypes: depressive type and manic type.

155 Which one of the following statements concerning the work of Sigmund Freud is correct?

   A. He believed transference to be vital in psychoanalysis.

   B. He initially listed nine neurotic defence mechanisms.

   C. Libido, Eros and Thanatos are important drives.

   D. The ego, superego and id are components of the Structural model.

   E. The oral, anal and phallic stages are components of the Topographical model.

156 Which of the following symptoms is not characteristic of temporal lobe epilepsy?

   A. Automatism.

   B. *Déjà vu.*

   C. Echolalia.

   D. Olfactory hallucinations.

   E. Pseudohallucinations.

153 **Answer: D.** Phobia is not a contraindication for dynamic psychotherapy; it is one of the indications. All other statements are correct. **[H. p. 354]**

154 **Answer: D.** DSM-IV schizoaffective disorder requires an uninterrupted period of illness in which both the A criteria for schizophrenia and for either a major depressive/mixed/manic episode are met. There must also have been at least two weeks in which there were psychotic symptoms without prominent mood symptoms. The minimum time period required to meet major depression criteria is two weeks, but mixed/manic episodes need just one week of symptoms. Since the A criteria for schizophrenia needs to be met (which require psychotic symptoms to be present for at least a month), the minimum period in which a schizoaffective episode can be diagnosed is one month. There are indeed two subtypes but these are the bipolar and depressive types. **[J. pp. 292–6]**

155 **Answer: C.** Freud considered transference to be a nuisance in therapy. His daughter Anna systematically listed nine defence mechanisms. Libido (sex drive), Eros (drive to preserve life) and Thanatos (death 'instinct') are the instinctual drives. The ego, superego and id are components of the Topographical model. The oral, anal and phallic stages are components of the Structural model. **[T. pp. 542–6; R. p. 164]**

156 **Answer: C.** Echolalia, the repetition of words or parts of sentences that are spoken in the patient's presence, more typically occurs in excited schizophrenic states, mental retardation and dementia. It is not part of the profile of temporal lobe epilepsy. An automatism is an action taking place in the absence of consciousness, and is characteristic of temporal lobe epilepsy. Pseudohallucinations may occur as autoscopy in temporal lobe epilepsy. *Déjà vu* and olfactory hallucinations can occur as part of the aura in temporal lobe epilepsy. Visual hallucinations may occur as part of the seizure. **[D. pp. 32, 88, 92, 95]**

157 A 63-year-old man, with a history of hypertension and carotid bruits bilaterally, presents to you for assessment of memory loss. He describes anxiety and trouble remembering names and dates. He has good insight into his memory loss and is aware that this loss of memory is of recent origin. Which psychiatric diagnosis is most likely in this case?

A. Alzheimer's dementia.

B. Frontal-lobe dementia.

C. Lewy-body dementia.

D. Normal pressure hydrocephalus.

E. Vascular dementia.

158 Which of the following is not a DSM-IV anxiety disorder?

A. Acute stress disorder.

B. Agoraphobia with panic disorder.

C. Post-traumatic stress disorder.

D. Social phobia.

E. Specific phobia.

159 Albert, who has paranoid schizophrenia, wants to know what might be the cause of his illness. From the list given below, which is the least likely cause for his illness?

A. Forceps delivery.

B. Birth in January.

C. Being born in London.

D. Having a brother with schizophrenia.

E. Strong family history of rheumatoid arthritis.

160 Freud described psychosexual stages. Which one of the following five choices lists them in the correct order?

A. Anal, Oral, Latent, Genital, Phallic.

B. Genital, Latent, Phallic, Anal, Oral.

C. Oral, Anal, Genital, Latent, Phallic.

D. Oral, Anal, Phallic, Latent, Genital.

E. Oral, Phallic, Anal, Latent, Genital.

157 **Answer: E.** Vascular dementia is the preferred diagnosis, as insight into the illness is present along with a more obvious onset than in Alzheimer's dementia. A cardiac history is also important; a step-wise progression in the course of the illness is described. Anxiety may also be present. **[G. pp. 410–12]**

158 **Answer: B.** ICD-10 and DSM-IV differ in their hierarchy of agoraphobia and panic disorder. Item B is an ICD-10 term: the DSM-IV equivalent would be panic disorder with agoraphobia. **[I. pp. 396–431]**

159 **Answer: E.** Rheumatoid arthritis is inversely related to the development of schizophrenia. All the other factors are environmental factors that contribute to the development of schizophrenia. **[AB. p. 190]**

160 **Answer: D.** This is the order of the psychosexual stages according to Freud. Failure to negotiate each stage coupled with the characteristic use of defence mechanisms may result in personality disorders. **[T. p. 546]**

161 A male patient with Tourette's syndrome is referred to the clinic for assessment. The referring doctor reports that in addition to vocal tics he has a number of other psychiatric difficulties associated with Tourette's syndrome. Which of the following symptoms is this patient least likely to display?

A. Anxiety.

B. Attention deficit.

C. Depression.

D. Obsessions.

E. Psychosis.

162 Aggression between children in the three to four-year-old age group is mirrored in primate species and takes which of the forms listed below?

A. Appeasement rituals.

B. Dominance hierarchies.

C. Fighting instinct.

D. Instrumental aggression.

E. Ritualisation.

163 Which of the following associations between neurotransmitters and sleep EEG is *not* correct?

A. Adrenergic stimulation and decreased REM sleep.

B. Cholinergic stimulation and wakefulness.

C. Dopaminergic activation and decreased REM sleep.

D. Histamine and active wakefulness.

E. Serotonergic activation and increased non-REM sleep.

164 Select the theorist below most closely associated with the following theory: *One's life is based upon satisfying various needs. At the most basic, these needs include essentials such as food and warmth. Once basic needs are met, individuals try to aim for higher needs such as love or respect. The highest level of need involves fulfilling one's full potential.*

A. Abraham Maslow.

B. Carl Rogers.

C. Frederick Perls.

D. Heinz Kohut.

E. Sandor Rado.

161 **Answer: E.** Patients with Tourette's syndrome have been found to have an increased prevalence of depression, anxiety and obsessional symptoms than normal controls. There is additionally an increased prevalence of deliberate self-harm. There does not appear to be any association with increased psychotic symptoms. **[D. p. 341; H. p. 287]**

162 **Answer: B.** Several species including primates form dominance hierarchies, where there is agreement on the status of animals within the group. Strayer described these dominance hierarchies among young children, where children with lower status within the group were less likely to show aggression to higher status children due to the hierarchy. Ethnologists studying animal behaviour described ritualisation and appeasement rituals. Ritualisation is aggression expressed in a stereotyped manner; hence injury or death is rare. Appeasement is surrender to avoid starting a fight in the first place. The fighting instinct was described by Lorenz and draws on Freud's psychodynamic model of aggression. Instrumental aggression is a distracter. **[C. pp. 100–3]**

163 **Answer: C.** Dopaminergic activation is associated with an increased REM sleep (not decreased); all other associations are correct. **[H. p. 212]**

164 **Answer: A.** What is being described is Maslow's hierarchy of need, with basic needs at the bottom of the pyramid and higher needs, such as self-actualisation, at the top. Needs such as security, belongingness and esteem come in-between on the hierarchy. **[F. pp. 78–9; P. p. 642]**

165 Margaret Mahler was an analyst who studied children and believed that they must pass through a sequence of maturational and developmental events in order to separate from the mother, and attain a stable sense of uniqueness. A child who successfully passed through the stages has hypothetically achieved which of the following?

A. Depressive position.

B. Object constancy.

C. Paranoid-schizoid position.

D. Separation-individuation.

E. Symbiosis.

166 A 55-year-old man presents with sudden onset unilateral facial paralysis. The upper and lower facial muscles are equally affected. The eyebrow droops and the wrinkles of the forehead are smoothed out. The muscles are equally affected for voluntary, emotional and associated movements. There is loss of taste on the anterior two-thirds of the tongue. The patient is well otherwise. Which of the following is the most likely diagnosis in this case?

A. Bell's palsy.

B. Horner's syndrome.

C. Multiple sclerosis.

D. Poliomyelitis.

E. Ramsay Hunt syndrome.

167 A three-year-old child attends for assessment. His parents are concerned that he rarely speaks; when he does, he appears to have adequate language for communication. There is no evidence of any problem with language comprehension or motor dysfunction. The child socialises well during the assessment. Which ICD-10 diagnosis is most likely in this case?

A. Asperger's syndrome.

B. Autism.

C. Elective mutism.

D. Receptive language disorder.

E. Rett's syndrome.

168 The term *demence precoce* is most associated with which author?

A. Benedict-Augustin Morel.

B. Emil Kraepelin.

C. Eugen Bleuler.

D. Gabriel Langfeldt.

E. Karl Jaspers.

165 **Answer: B.** The depressive and paranoid-schizoid positions are Kleinian concepts. Separation and Symbiosis are the first two of Mahler's developmental stages and the third stage is 'on the road to object constancy'. **[T. p. 551]**

166 **Answer: A.** Bell's palsy is diagnosed by the sudden onset of a unilateral facial paralysis with or without loss of taste in the anterior two-thirds of the tongue in a person who is otherwise well. Ramsay Hunt syndrome occurs with herpes zoster of the geniculate ganglia: there is a facial palsy identical to Bell's palsy but with herpetic lesions in the external auditory meatus. Deafness may occur. Multiple sclerosis should be considered as a possible cause when unilateral facial paralysis occurs in a young adult, especially if it is painless, not very severe and clears up in two or three weeks. Poliomyelitis should be considered as a cause when unilateral facial paralysis occurs during an epidemic of that disease especially in a child or adolescent and if it occurs a few days after a febrile illness. **[AL. pp. 67–9; AK. p. 888]**

167 **Answer: C.** Elective mutism is the most likely diagnosis. Autism is excluded due to not having any restricted, repetitive behaviours and having normal social interactions, although there are communication difficulties. There is no evidence of receptive language problems as comprehension is intact in this case. Rett's syndrome occurs only in girls. **[I. pp. 232–59]**

168 **Answer: A.** Kraepelin changed Morel's term to *dementia praecox* while Bleuler used the term *schizophrenia*. Langfeldt is associated with *schizophreniform psychosis*. **[F. p. 79; P. pp. 1170–1]**

169 A patient has been prescribed chlorpromazine for the last year. He describes getting a rash on his body whenever he sits in the sunshine. Which of the following best describes this side-effect of chlorpromazine?

A. Anti-adrenergic side-effect.

B. Anticholinergic side-effect.

C. Antihistaminic side-effect.

D. Extra-pyramidal side-effect.

E. Idiosyncratic side-effect.

170 Donald Winnicott was a British paediatrician interested in object relations who developed many psychoanalytic concepts. Which of the following is not one of them?

A. At-one-ment.

B. Going on being.

C. Good-enough mother.

D. Good breast.

E. Transitional object.

171 A 36-year-old woman who was diagnosed with puerperal psychosis attends the outpatient department accompanied by her husband. They would like to have more children but want to know what the chances are of the illness recurring. Which of the following figures best represents this woman's chance of becoming psychotic again following childbirth?

A. 1%.

B. 5%.

C. 10%.

D. 20%.

E. 30%.

172 A 25-year-old woman suffering with a depressive episode has a night of complete insomnia. Which of the symptoms below is she most likely to display?

A. Daytime somnolence.

B. Improvement in her depressive symptoms.

C. Mania.

D. Unchanged mood.

E. Worsening of her depressive symptoms.

169 **Answer: E.** Other idiosyncratic side-effects of chlorpromazine include: cholestatic jaundice, altered glucose tolerance, hypersensitivity reactions and skin photosensitivity. **[AB. pp. 210–11]**

170 **Answer: D.** The 'good breast' is a Kleinian concept. **[R. p. 166]**

171 **Answer: E.** Women who experience a puerperal psychosis have a one in three chance of a further psychotic episode following a subsequent pregnancy. This woman's risk would be further increased by a personal or family history of a major mental disorder. Risk is higher in women with a history of bipolar rather than unipolar affective disorder. **[A. p. 560]**

172 **Answer: B.** An improvement in mood is the best answer in this case. Sleep deprivation is used in mood disorders for several reasons, including augmenting the response to antidepressant medication, or as an antidepressant in treatment-resistant depression. It takes several forms, i.e. total sleep deprivation, or late partial sleep deprivation. **[G. p. 216]**

173 A pseudo-seizure (non-epileptic attack) is an unlikely diagnosis in which of the following situations?

A. If it happens following an emotional precipitant.

B. If it happens outdoors.

C. If it happens when others are present.

D. If serum prolactin is not raised after the attack.

E. If the patient talks or screams during the attack.

174 Select the theorist below most closely associated with the following theory: *The individual develops specific behavioural traits to defend against threats both from within the individual and without. This character armour prevents repressed impulses from being acted upon. They may translate into physical manifestations such as specific postures or movements for the individual.*

A. Erich Fromm.   B. Harry Stack Sullivan.

C. Karen Horney.   D. Otto Rank.

E. Wilhelm Reich.

175 The terms *inferiority complex* and *sibling rivalry* are associated with which of the following psychoanalysts?

A. Alfred Adler.   B. Anna Freud.

C. Karen Horney.   D. Sigmund Freud.

E. Wilfred Bion.

176 A 22-year-old woman has been referred for the neurology service for assessment. She was initially referred to a neurologist for treatment of seizures. However, the neurologist is of the opinion that she is not experiencing true seizures. Which of the following features would suggest that this woman is presenting with non-epileptic seizures?

A. Extensor plantar reflexes following the seizure.

B. Incontinence.

C. Increased seizure activity when attempts are made to restrain the patient.

D. Loss of corneal reflexes during and following the seizure.

E. Tonic-clonic seizures.

173 **Answer: B.** Pseudo-seizures most commonly occur indoors at home. They are also associated with the other circumstances listed in the items. **[H. p. 205]**

174 **Answer: E.** Reich's theory of personality development is still influential because of the utility of the concept of *character armour*. His ideas on how this can translate into body posture and so on have been less regarded, however. **[P. pp. 627–8]**

175 **Answer: A.** Alfred Adler was a neo-Freudian and emphasised the importance of social factors in development. He was a key figure in the development of group-based therapies. **[T. pp. 547–8]**

176 **Answer: C.** Non-epileptic seizures occur commonly in patients who also experience epileptic seizures. The movements in non-epileptic seizures often involve generalised rigidity with arching of the back and random thrashing of the limbs, contrasting with the stereotypical tonic-clonic movements in grand mal seizures. Reflexes are unaltered in non-epileptic attacks. Incontinence is common in epileptic seizures but rare in non-epileptic episodes. **[A. p. 318]**

177 Which of the following factors optimise patients' compliance with medication?

A. Increased dosage frequency.

B. Multiple pills per day.

C. Medication with troublesome side-effects.

D. Oral medication.

E. Patient education.

178 The description of the antidepressant effects of imipramine is most associated with whom of the following?

A. Egas Moniz.

B. John Cade.

C. Paul Charpentier.

D. Roland Kuhn.

E. Ugo Cerletti.

179 James has recently been diagnosed with schizophrenia. His mother is anxious about him and asks you about his long-term prognosis. Which of the following features is the worst prognostic factor?

A. Acute sudden onset.

B. Having a family member with bipolar disorder.

C. Late onset.

D. Negative symptoms of schizophrenia.

E. Paranoid delusions.

180 Which one of the following is not a feature of brief dynamic psychotherapy?

A. A focus on the link between the present problem, the past and the therapeutic relationship.

B. A focus on the termination of therapy from the start.

C. Passive therapist style.

D. Time limited.

E. Triangle of person.

177 **Answer: E.** Decreased dosage and lower frequency of medication opti-mise compliance. So too does patient and family education and parenteral rather than oral medication. Clear labelling and use of medication that is well tolerated with few side-effects is optimal for patient concordance. **[G. p. 157]**

178 **Answer: D.** All those listed were pioneers in psychiatric physical thera-pies. Kuhn reported the antidepressant properties of imipramine in 1957. Moniz is associated with psychosurgery, Cade with the descrip-tion of the mood-stabilising effects of lithium and Charpentier with the antipsychotic properties of chlorpromazine. Cerletti, with his colleague Lucio Bini, described the effects of electroconvulsive therapy. **[F. p. 78; P. p. 2491]**

179 **Answer: D.** Negative symptoms of schizophrenia are considered a sign of poor prognosis. Similarly, simple schizophrenia is believed to have a poor prognosis. All the other factors confer good prognosis. **[AB. p. 185]**

180 **Answer: C.** The therapist is active in brief dynamic psychotherapy. **[T. p. 555]**

181 A patient reports that he has been experiencing visual hallucinations. He describes seeing the face of his sister in the pattern on his kitchen floor tiles. Which of the following perceptual abnormalities is this man experiencing?

A. Affect illusion.

B. Completion illusion.

C. Elementary hallucination.

D. Functional hallucination.

E. Pareidolic illusion.

182 The strength of the placebo effect in the treatment of anxiety is strongest in which of the following physical forms of medication?

A. Capsule.

B. Yellow colour medication.

C. Single pill.

D. Small pill.

E. Tablet.

183 Regarding early psychoanalytic theorists, which of the following pairings is not correct?

A. Alfred Adler and individual psychology.

B. Anna Freud and defence mechanisms.

C. Carl Jung and archetypes.

D. Karen Horney and psychobiology.

E. Melanie Klein and object relations.

184 Choose the most correct statement regarding stigma and mental health:

A. In Europe northern countries are more tolerant of mental illness.

B. Nowadays the media has an overall positive view of mental illness.

C. The closure of asylums has reduced stigma towards mental illness.

D. The lack of objective markers of mental illness reduces stigma.

E. The public feels antidepressants are the best treatment for depression.

181 **Answer: E.** There are three types of illusion. A completion illusion occurs when an incomplete perception that is meaningless in itself is filled in a process of extrapolation from previous experience to produce significance. An affect illusion is one which can be understood in the context of the person's mood state, for example when a child frightened by the dark mistakes a blowing curtain for a person in the room. Pareidolic illusions are created out of sensory percepts by an admixture with imagination. Functional hallucinations occur when a certain percept is necessary for the production of a hallucination but the hallucination is not a transformation of that percept. For example, the patient hears voices when a tap is turned on. An elementary hallucination is an auditory hallucination of unstructured sounds, often occurring in an organic state. **[D. pp. 81–5]**

182 **Answer: A.** Patients with anxiety disorders responded better to green-coloured medication, patients with depressive disorders to yellow tablets. These pill factors are related to placebo strength: multiple pills are greater than single pills and larger pills are greater than smaller pills. Capsules have greater strength than tablets. **[G. p. 158]**

183 **Answer: D.** Adolf Meyer is associated with psychobiology. Karen Horney is associated with holistic psychology and basic anxiety. **[F. pp. 71–7]**

184 **Answer: A.** Northern European countries tend to be more tolerant, although southern European countries may have more family supports. Some studies have found the media still has an overall negative view of mental illness. Lack of objective markers for mental illness can have the effect of allowing some to believe that such illness is 'made up'. The public often has concerns regarding potential addictiveness of antidepressants: 'counselling' is generally felt by the lay public to be the best treatment for depression. The closure of asylums has helped stigma in some regards, but it has also increased fears in some countries regarding dangerousness of patients in the community. Thus while C is partially true, A is the 'most correct'. **[M. pp. 5–8, 1534–5]**

185 Reformulation, recognise, revision, dilemmas, traps and snags are terms associated with which psychotherapy?

A. Brief dynamic psychotherapy.

B. Cognitive analytic therapy.

C. Cognitive behaviour therapy.

D. Interpersonal therapy.

E. Solution focused therapy.

186 A 25-year-old woman is referred for assessment by the obstetric SHO. She is reported to be feeling depressed following the birth of her first baby three days ago. She has no previous history of depression. The baby is healthy, although the woman required a Caesarean section to deliver. Which of the following is the most likely diagnosis?

A. Adjustment disorder.

B. Adjustment reaction.

C. Baby blues.

D. Major depression with post-partum onset.

E. Major depressive disorder.

187 A 25-year-old woman who was sexually abused as a young child and now as an adult has no memory of being abused is using which Freudian defence mechanism from the list below?

A. Incorporation.

B. Isolation.

C. Rationalisation.

D. Repression.

E. Undoing.

188 Which of the following is a risk factor for antidepressant-induced hyponatraemia?

A. Being overweight.

B. Cold weather.

C. Impaired renal function.

D. Male sex.

E. Younger age.

185 **Answer: B.** Cognitive analytic therapy was developed by Ryle and is an example of a brief dynamic psychotherapy. Interpersonal therapy was developed for depressed patients and focuses on interpersonal relationships. Solution focused therapy is a branch of strategic family therapy. **[T. p. 556; W. p. 242]**

186 **Answer: C.** Baby blues typically occurs three to six days following the birth of the baby in 50–60% of mothers. Post-partum depression occurs in approximately 10% of women post partum. It usually occurs within six to eight weeks of birth, most often beginning between day 3 and 14 post partum. Adjustment disorder is usually diagnosed within six months of the occurrence of a significant stressor, and usually resolves within six months of the resolution of the stressful situation. An adjustment reaction is a short-lived anxiety response to a stressful situation. Given the time frame of this presentation, the birth and the prevalence, the most likely diagnosis is baby blues. **[H. pp. 380–1; AH. pp. 285–6]**

187 **Answer: D.** Repression is the basic defence of pushing something away. In this case, if successful, no memory will be left in the conscious mind. Rationalisation is an attempt to explain in a logically consistent manner thoughts and feelings whose true motives are not perceived. **[G. p. 103]**

188 **Answer: C.** Older age, female sex, low body weight and warm weather are risk factors. Other risk factors include impaired renal function, some other medical conditions (such as hypertension) and co-administration of some drugs (e.g. carbamazepine). **[V. pp. 210–11]**

189 A patient who was admitted involuntarily to hospital for relapse of paranoid schizophrenia improved one month after his admission. Nursing staff have noticed, however, that he is pacing around a lot in the corridor. While you want to interview him to see whether he is relapsing he tells you that he finds it difficult to stay in one position. What would be the most appropriate line of treatment that you might try in order to relieve his symptoms?

A. Add in a low dose of olanzapine.

B. Add in a low dose of risperidone.

C. Reassure him and review him again in one week's time.

D. Start him on a benzodiazepine.

E. Start him on a selective serotonin reuptake inhibitor (SSRI).

190 Bateman, Brown and Pedder list four selection criteria when considering which patients should be offered level-three psychotherapy. Which of the following is not one of them?

A. They are able to form and maintain relationships.

B. They have a problem understandable in psychological terms.

C. They have at least average intelligence.

D. They have sufficient motivation for insight and change.

E. They have the requisite ego strength.

191 A 22-year-old man with schizophrenia is an inpatient on the psychiatric ward. Nursing staff request that he be reviewed urgently. He is sweating and confused. On examination he has severe rigidity, tachycardia, and his blood pressure is fluctuating. His temperature is 106°F. He has been treated with aripiprazole. Which of the following is the most likely diagnosis in this case?

A. Catatonia.   B. Delirium.

C. Myocardial infarct.   D. Neuroleptic malignant syndrome.

E. Tetanus.

192 A 15-year-old boy with a diagnosis of obsessive compulsive disorder (OCD) touches the tap in the bathroom of his home three times after thinking a distressing thought about being contaminated by germs. What is the prominent defence mechanism displayed by this boy in touching the tap?

A. Isolation.   B. Rationalisation.

C. Reaction formation.   D. Reversal into the opposite.

E. Undoing.

189 **Answer: D.** This man is suffering from akathisia, i.e. a subjective feeling of restlessness usually of the lower limbs, which most commonly occurs with typical antipsychotics prescribed for more than one month. The usual treatment is with a reduction of antipsychotic dose, change to an atypical agent (not just add one in) or by adding propranolol or a benzodiazepine. **[V. pp. 92–3]**

190 **Answer: C.** Intelligence is not one of the criteria. **[T. p. 554]**

191 **Answer: D.** The diagnosis of neuroleptic malignant syndrome (NMS) requires rigidity and elevated temperature in a patient on antipsychotic medication. The onset may be gradual or rapid, and most typically occurs in a young male recently commenced on neuroleptics. There are case reports in the literature of NMS occurring with aripiprazole. Catatonia may present with rigidity, but is not accompanied by pyrexia or signs of autonomic instability. Tetanus presents with muscular spasm usually beginning in the masseter muscle and generalising. It is accompanied by autonomic dysfunction but the patient is mentally alert. Delirium presents with confusion of varying degrees, and may be accompanied by pyrexia though not by rigidity. Myocardial infarction may present with hypotension, diaphoresis and tachycardia, but will be marked by severe chest pain; there will be no rigidity. **[V. pp. 103–5]**

192 **Answer: E.** Undoing is an attempt to atone for or negate a forbidden thought, affect or memory. In this case a thought regarding contamination is being magically undone by touching the tap. Isolation and reaction formation are the two other defence mechanisms used in OCD. **[G. p. 103]**

193 All of the following are part of Yalom's curative factors except:
   A. Altruism.
   B. Empathy.
   C. Existential factors.
   D. Group cohesiveness.
   E. Interpersonal learning.

194 The community psychiatric nurse asks you to review a 24-year-old girl earlier than scheduled in your outpatient clinic. She has marked anxiety symptoms, irritability, sweating, impaired sleep and paraesthesia. It turns out she stopped her antidepressant herself two days earlier. Which antidepressant is most likely to have caused her symptoms?
   A. Citalopram.
   B. Fluoxetine.
   C. Mirtazapine.
   D. Sertraline.
   E. Venlafaxine.

195 The behavioural therapy whereby a patient is exposed to an anxiety-provoking stimulus to decrease arousal is known as?
   A. Graded exposure.
   B. Habituation.
   C. Reciprocal inhibition.
   D. Shaping.
   E. Systematic desensitisation.

196 A 35-year-old woman is referred to your clinic from another psychiatry service. She is initially cross that she is not seeing the consultant. In recounting her employment history she reports that she worked for a very prominent firm but was overlooked for promotion on a number of occasions and left. She believes that others in her department conspired to prevent her promotion as they were jealous of her potential. She reports that she is currently seeking another position but feels that she is overqualified for the positions available. She says that she finds it difficult to befriend women as they are often envious of her. She reports that she is currently in a wonderful relationship, which she says began two weeks previously. She says that her new partner is an airline pilot. She asks if you could make an exception and see her in the evening time as she is quite busy during the day and doesn't like to have to sit in the outpatients department. What is the most likely diagnosis in this case?
   A. Borderline personality disorder.
   B. Histrionic personality disorder.
   C. Narcissistic personality disorder.
   D. Paranoid personality disorder.
   E. Schizotypal personality disorder.

193 **Answer: B.** Empathy is not one of Yalom's curative factors. The other factors include: catharsis, group cohesiveness, development of socialising techniques and imitative behaviour. **[M. p. 1448]**

194 **Answer: E.** While many antidepressants can cause a discontinuation syndrome, venlafaxine has the most potential to cause it from this list (fluoxetine has the least because of its long half-life). Other antidepressants particularly associated with a discontinuation syndrome include paroxetine, amitriptyline, imipramine and the MAOIs. **[V. pp. 240–3]**

195 **Answer: B.** However, the other items are all aspects of behavioural therapy for phobias where it is presumed that the phobia is a conditioned fear response to a stimulus. **[T. p. 566]**

196 **Answer: C.** This woman demonstrates the following traits of narcissistic personality disorder:
- a grandiose sense of self-importance
- a sense of entitlement
- believes that others are envious of her
- believes that she is special and unique and can only be understood by other special or high-status people
- requires excessive admiration.

She has traits of other personality disorders:
- Histrionic personality disorder: considers relationships to be more intimate than they actually are.
- Borderline personality disorder: a pattern of unstable and intense interpersonal relationships.
- Her concern regarding her former colleagues is more a rationalisation of her failure to meet her own expectations than a pervasive distrust or suspiciousness as in a paranoid personality disorder. While she appears to lack friendships she does not meet other criteria for a schizotypal personality disorder. **[AH. pp. 287–97]**

197 A 30-year-old male cyclist is hit by a car while crossing a junction. He suffers a head injury with loss of consciousness as a result. Which is the gravest prognostic indicator listed below?

A. Anterograde amnesia of less than 12 hours.

B. Closed skull fracture.

C. No amnesia symptoms.

D. Penetrating skull fracture.

E. Retrograde amnesia less than one hour.

198 A 32-year-old woman with depression has been prescribed a hypnotic by her general practitioner. When she wakes in the morning she feels groggy for an hour or two. Which hypnotic was she most likely prescribed?

A. Promethazine.

B. Temazepam.

C. Zaleplon.

D. Zopiclone.

E. Zolpidem.

199 Mrs Knox has recently been diagnosed with depression. She wants to know about the long-term outcome of her illness. From the list below, which one is a good prognostic factor in her case?

A. Endogenous depression.

B. Insidious onset.

C. Neurotic depression.

D. Personality disorder.

E. Residual symptoms.

200 In cognitive behaviour therapy (CBT) the cognitive distortion whereby a patient attends solely to the negative aspects of a situation is known as?

A. Arbitrary inference.

B. Dichotomous thinking.

C. Negative automatic thoughts.

D. Schema.

E. Selective abstraction.

197 **Answer: D.** A penetrating head injury has a poorer prognosis than a closed head injury. Anterograde amnesia of 12 hours or less usually has a good prognosis with no long-term sequelae. Retrograde amnesia is not a good prognostic indicator of clinical course. **[H. p. 193]**

198 **Answer: A.** This hang-over effect is related to the duration of action: from the list promethazine has the longest. Promethazine is not licensed as a hypnotic and has a relatively prolonged period between taking the tablet and falling asleep (up to one to two hours). From the list, the hypnotic with the next longest duration of action is zopiclone. **[V. p. 269]**

199 **Answer: A.** Endogenous depression has a better outcome than neurotic depression. Other good prognostic factors are acute onset and earlier age of onset. All the other symptoms given are poor prognostic factors. **[AB. p. 258]**

200 **Answer: E.** Arbitrary inference means 'jumping to conclusions'. Dichotomous thinking means 'all or nothing' or 'black and white' thinking. The identification and evaluation of negative automatic thoughts is central to CBT. Schemas are the deeply held beliefs which give rise to our personality and may be the target of later therapy. **[W. p. 174]**

201 A 42-year-old man presents for assessment, having been transferred from another service. He tells you that he has 'manic depression'. Which of the following phenomena would most lead you to doubt this diagnosis?

A. Delusional mood.

B. Delusional perception.

C. Delusions of persecution.

D. Flight of ideas.

E. Voices talking to the patient.

202 The rivalry between a son and his father for his mother's affection in Freudian psychoanalysis is best described by which of the terms described below?

A. Castration anxiety.

B. Electra complex.

C. Oedipal complex.

D. Oral envy.

E. Oral frustration.

203 In a 50-year-old patient with a head injury who seeks compensation, which of the following is less likely to contribute to long-term disability?

A. Female sex.

B. Financial compensation is possible.

C. Industrial injury.

D. Low social status.

E. The patient feels that someone else is at fault.

204 In relation to contribution of predisposing life events and difficulties to depression in adulthood, which of the factors below has not been proposed as an aetiological factor?

A. Having three or more children under the age of 14 years.

B. Lack of a close confidant.

C. Loss of father by age 11 from separation or death.

D. Not working outside the home.

E. None of the above answers is incorrect.

201 **Answer: B.** Delusional perception is a first-rank symptom of schizophrenia. Delusional mood is considered not to be restricted to people with schizophrenia, but is also noted in affective disorders such as puerperal depression. While first-rank symptoms can occur in bipolar disorder, they should always make one consider schizophrenia. **[D. pp. 110, 149–54]**

202 **Answer: C.** The Electra complex is the female equivalent of the Oedipal complex. Castration anxiety in males resolves the Oedipal complex. Oral envy and frustration are from Kleinian theory and are stages in development of the child during the first year of development. **[G. p. 101; H. p. 335]**

203 **Answer: A.** The listed items are compensation issues that are more likely to contribute to disability with the exception of sex: being male and having compensation issues is more likely to lead to disability. **[H. p. 195]**

204 **Answer: C.** The original Brown and Harris Camberwell family study mentions four main life difficulties and predisposing life events as significant aetiological factors for depression in adult life. They are: not working outside the home, lack of close confidant and intimacy, having three or more children all under the age 14 years and, finally, loss of a child's mother (not father as in option C) from death or separation. The presence of childhood adversity, e.g. sexual and physical abuse, has been subsequently implicated. **[AG. pp. 216–17]**

205 Which one of the following inhibits the cytochrome p450 system and therefore causes a clinically important increase in the plasma level of clozapine?

A. Carbamazepine.

B. Fluvoxamine.

C. Smoking.

D. Sodium valproate.

E. Warfarin.

206 A 45-year-old man attends for assessment. He has been transferred from another service and you have been told that he has a diagnosis of schizophrenia. Which of the following symptoms would provide the weakest evidence for this diagnosis?

A. Delusional perception.

B. Delusions of passivity.

C. Delusions of persecution.

D. Third-party auditory hallucinations.

E. Thought broadcasting.

207 A 53-year-old man who believes that his stomach has rotted away and he should not eat because he has no stomach has which syndrome below?

A. Cotard's syndrome.

B. Couvade syndrome.

C. Ekbom's syndrome.

D. Ganser syndrome.

E. Othello syndrome.

208 Which one of the people mentioned below is most closely associated with learned helplessness as a model for aetiology of depression?

A. Aaron Beck.

B. Anton Mesmer.

C. Martin Seligman.

D. Melanie Klein.

E. Wilfred Bion.

205 **Answer: B.** Carbamazepine induces the metabolism of clozapine (3A4). Fluvoxamine inhibits cytochrome p450 1A2 and increases the level of clozapine. Smoking induces the p450 system (1A2). Sodium valproate may decrease clozapine levels. **[AI. pp. 235, 298–301]**

206 **Answer: C.** Delusions of persecution are a non-specific psychotic symptom. All other options are first-rank symptoms of schizophrenia. **[D. pp. 149–54]**

207 **Answer: A.** Cotard's syndrome is commoner in females and involves nihilistic delusions usually of their body or self having disappeared. Couvade syndrome is where the husband develops anxiety along with several symptoms of pregnancy, during his wife's pregnancy. Ekbom's syndrome is a delusion of infestation with insects. Ganser syndrome is described as the 'syndrome of approximate answers'. **[H. pp. 163–6, D. p. 123]**

208 **Answer: C.** Martin Seligman proposed the concept of learned helplessness. He drew a parallel between animal models (where the animal is unable to control or escape from persistently punishing stimuli) and human models of depression. Aaron Beck is associated with depressive cognitions and cognitive distortions in depression. Melanie Klein is associated with object-relations theory and the paranoid and depressive positions. Anton Mesmer is associated with animal magnetism and hypnosis. Wilfred Bion is associated with group psychotherapy. **[AU. pp. 218–19, 603, 615]**

209 A man has recently been diagnosed with bipolar affective disorder. He asks you how likely it is that his brothers or sisters may get the same illness. From your knowledge of the genetic role in the aetiology of bipolar affective disorder, what answer would you choose from the following?

A. Fifteen times.

B. No extra risk.

C. Seven times.

D. Ten times.

E. Three times.

210 Which one of the following is true concerning the antipsychotic clozapine?

A. It causes a fatal agranulocytosis in 0.1% of patients.

B. It causes neutropaenia in 0.7% of patients.

C. It is a $5HT_2$ agonist.

D. It is 95% protein bound.

E. It is primarily a D_2 blocker.

211 Which of the following drugs is least likely to cause serotonin syndrome?

A. Ecstasy.

B. Fluoxetine.

C. Olanzapine.

D. Phenelzine.

E. Venlafaxine.

212 A 23-year-old man presents for the first time to your psychiatric service with a three-month history of hearing third-person auditory hallucinations. On which of the criteria below would he not be diagnosed with schizophrenia?

A. Catego.

B. DSM-IV.

C. Feighner's criteria.

D. ICD-10.

E. Research Diagnostic Criteria.

209 **Answer: C.** First-degree relatives are seven times more likely to develop the condition when compared to other people. Monozygotic twins have 33–90% risk of developing bipolar affective disorder when compared to dizygotic twins who have a risk of approximately 23%. **[AB. p. 310]**

210 **Answer: D.** Clozapine causes neutropenia in 2.7% of patients, and fatal agranulocytosis in less than 0.01% of patients. It is a $5HT_{2A}$ antagonist and has comparatively low D_2 affinity (but high D_4 affinity). **[V. pp. 75–7]**

211 **Answer: C.** Olanzapine is not associated with serotonin syndrome. The other drugs have all been implicated in serotonin syndrome. Ecstasy has been associated with serotonin syndrome in combination with venlafaxine. **[X. pp. 372–3]**

212 **Answer: C.** Feighner's criteria requires six months' duration of illness for diagnosis, while the Research Diagnostic Criteria requires at least two weeks' duration of illness. ICD-10 requires one month. DSM-IV requires one month or less if successfully treated. In Catego a computerised algorithm generated from the Present State Examination takes no account of duration. **[H. pp. 27–8]**

213 Which of the following is not a part of client-centred therapy?

A. Accurate empathy.

B. Basic encounters.

C. Genuineness.

D. Permissiveness.

E. Unconditional positive regard.

214 Which of the options below least supports the monoamine hypothesis of depression?

A. Blunting of growth hormone response to clonidine and desipramine.

B. Dexamethasone non-suppression of endogenous cortisol.

C. Increase in cortical 5-HT$_2$ receptor binding.

D. Reduced 5-HIAA concentration in CSF of suicide attempters.

E. Reduction in CSF HVA concentration.

215 A patient recently commenced on clozapine titration has a resting tachycardia of 102 bpm. You should:

A. Cease clozapine.

B. Prescribe a beta-blocker.

C. Prescribe an anticholinergic.

D. Refer promptly to the cardiology team.

E. Slow down the titration and decrease the dose if needed.

216 A woman is pregnant with her first child. Her father had schizophrenia. She is afraid that her child will develop schizophrenia in later life. Which figure best represents her child's lifetime risk of developing schizophrenia?

A. 1%.

B. 5%.

C. 15%.

D. 20%.

E. 50%.

213 **Answer: D.** Permissiveness is one of the basic features for therapeutic communities according to Rapoport. Rogers' client-centred therapy involves: genuineness, unconditional positive regard, accurate empathy and non-directive acceptance. **[H. pp. 358–61]**

214 **Answer: B.** Non-suppression of endogenous cortisol following dexamethasone challenge has been demonstrated as a hypothalamic-pituitary-adrenal axis derangement in depression. The three main neurotransmitter systems implicated in the monoamine hypothesis of depression are 5-HT, noradrenaline and dopamine. Clonidine, a noradrenaline receptor agonist and desipramine, a noradrenaline re-uptake antagonist, act to increase plasma growth hormone concentration. A blunting of this response may be seen in depression. Homovanilic acid (HVA) is a breakdown product of dopamine. It has been less consistently shown to be reduced in post-mortem studies of depressed patients. 5-hydroxyindoleacetic acid (5-HIAA), the main metabolite of 5-HT, is significantly reduced in the CSF of suicide attempters. $5-HT_2$ receptor binding reflects an adaptive up-regulation in $5-HT_2$ receptor population. This is an adaptive mechanism following reduction in pre-synaptic 5-HT production which may be observed in depression. **[M. pp. 181–7]**

215 **Answer: E.** This is probably mediated by clozapine's antimuscarinic action and tends to respond to reducing the dose and slowing the titration. If it doesn't settle, prescribing a beta-blocker may help. Anticholinergics would increase the heart rate. Myocarditis should be suspected if the tachycardia is accompanied by chest pain, ECG changes, heart failure, and influenza-like symptoms. **[V. p. 70]**

216 **Answer: B.** The grandchild of a person with schizophrenia has a 5% lifetime risk of developing the illness. The sibling of a patient where one of the parents has schizophrenia has a risk of 17%, as does the dizygotic twin of a person with schizophrenia. The monozygotic twin of a patient with schizophrenia or the child of two parents with schizophrenia has a risk of almost 50% of developing the illness. **[S. p. 275]**

217 A 22-year-old mother of two children with a history of recurrent depressive disorder presents to you with thoughts of ending her life. Which of the questions below is the most significant in her risk assessment?

A. History of pessimistic views of the future.

B. History of reduced appetite.

C. History of reduced concentration.

D. History of sleep disturbance.

E. History of thought of harm to her children.

218 A 36-year-old man with depression reports to you: 'I lost my last job, so I must be useless and a bad person. Life is not worth living anymore'. What defence mechanism is this man using at this point?

A. Introjection.

B. Passive death wish.

C. Projective self-harm.

D. Reality confrontation.

E. Turning against the self.

219 A cardiology registrar rings you about a patient who is on lithium therapy. He has recently done an ECG and has found some abnormal changes. From the list below, select which one is the ECG change that can be caused by lithium:

A. Absent P wave.

B. Atrial fibrillation.

C. Depression of the ST segment.

D. Elevation of the ST segment.

E. Flattening of the T wave.

220 Risperidone is a:

A. Aliphatic phenothiazine.

B. Benzisoxazole.

C. Butyrophenone.

D. Dibenzothiazepine.

E. Thienobenzodiazepine.

217 **Answer: E.** Symptoms A to D are common in depressive illness. In a parent with depressive illness, it is essential to check regarding risk to their children. **[I. p. 119]**

218 **Answer: E.** Turning against the self is an ego defence mechanism seen in depression. It was initially espoused in Freud's *Mourning and Melancholia*. The individual turns unacceptable impulses and aggression towards others to himself. Introjection is an immature defence in which the qualities of an external object are internalised and subsequently identified with. The rest are not ego defence mechanisms. **[S. pp. 220, 556–7]**

219 **Answer: E.** T wave flattening is caused by lithium and also widening of QRS complexes. These are benign ECG changes related to lithium therapy. Rarely, lithium can also exacerbate existing arrhythmias or new arrhythmias due to conduction deficits at the SA or AV nodes. **[AB. p. 330]**

220 **Answer: B.** Examples of the other groups are as follows: aliphatic phenothiazine – chlorpromazine; butyrophenone – haloperidol; dibenzothiazepine – quetiapine; thienobenzodiazepine – olanzapine. **[E. pp. 2360, 2457]**

221 Which of the following disorders is least likely to be an underlying cause of depression?

A. Acromegaly.

B. Addison's disease.

C. Cushing's syndrome.

D. Hyperparathyroidism.

E. Hypothyroidism.

222 A 24-year-old male on his first presentation to your psychiatric service is admitted with a history of mania. He is one week on the acute unit and his mood remains elated. Your consultant asks you to use a rating scale to quantify his symptoms. Which of the following rating scales would you use?

A. Beck inventory.

B. McGill questionnaire.

C. Yale-Brown scale.

D. Young scale.

E. Zung scale.

223 Basic features of therapeutic communities according to Rapoport include the following, except:

A. Communalism.

B. Democratisation.

C. Permissiveness.

D. Reality confrontation.

E. Self-actualisation.

224 The following are processes in family therapy, except:

A. Circular questioning in systemic family therapy.

B. Childhood projective systems and unconscious conflicts in psychodynamic family therapy.

C. Homework assignments in psychodynamic family therapy.

D. Analysis of family rules and relationships in structural family therapy.

E. The use of paradoxical injunction in systemic family therapy.

221 **Answer: A.** Diseases of the glucocorticoid axis (Addison's and Cushing's syndromes) and of the thyroid axis may present with depression as a symptom. A recent study found no increase in depression levels in acromegaly compared with the general population. **[AK. pp. 800–16; Abed RT, Clark J, Elbadawy MHF, Cliffe MJ. Psychiatric morbidity in acromegaly.** *Acta Psychiatrica Scandinavica.* **2007; 75: 635–9]**

222 **Answer: D.** The Young Mania Rating Scale is an 11-item observer rated scale. The Beck Depression Inventory is a self-rating depression scale with 21 items. The Zung Anxiety Scale is a 20-item, combined observer and self-report. The Yale-Brown Obsessive Compulsive Scale is an observer-rated 19-item scale. The McGill Pain Questionnaire is a self-report questionnaire. **[H. p. 7]**

223 **Answer: E.** Self-actualisation is one of Maslow's stages of basic human needs, while the other options in this question are the four basic features of therapeutic communities according to Rapoport. **[H. p. 361]**

224 **Answer: C.** *Homework assignments* are used in cognitive behaviour therapy: it is not a process in family therapy. The rest are indeed processes used in the respective types of family therapies mentioned. In psychodynamic family therapy, unconscious conflicts may lead to family difficulties. *Childhood projective systems* are adult expectations that have a basis in childhood experiences. These experiences guide relationships between parents and also their relationships with their children. **[E. pp. 2157–67, 2821–31]**

225 A patient's serum lithium (12 hours post last dose) is 3.0 mmol/L. Which one of the following is a sign of lithium toxicity?

A. Coarse tremor.

B. Fine tremor.

C. Hair loss.

D. Photophobia.

E. Polydipsia.

226 In the classification of personality disorders which of the following disorders has diagnostic criteria listed in DSM-IV but not in ICD-10?

A. Dependent personality disorder.

B. Histrionic personality disorder.

C. Narcissistic personality disorder.

D. Schizoid personality disorder.

E. Schizotypal disorder.

227 A 29-year-old patient with a seven-year history of schizophrenia attends your psychiatric service. He lives with his parents and has described to you receiving numerous critical comments from his parents. He reports that they are hostile towards him at times. Which of the interventions listed below would be most beneficial in this case?

A. Cognitive remediation.

B. Cognitive behaviour therapy.

C. Family therapy.

D. Social skills training.

E. Treatment as usual.

228 A 14-year-old girl still carries around a piece of her mother's clothing since her early childhood. She claims that this item of clothing comforts and reminds her of her mother, who is baffled at this persisting behaviour. Who is most closely associated with the description of this phenomenon?

A. Alfred Adler.

B. Carl Jung.

C. Carl Rogers.

D. Donald Winnicott.

E. Erik Erikson.

225 **Answer: A.** Hair loss is not a sign of toxicity of lithium but can be an adverse effect. Photophobia is not associated with lithium toxicity. Polyuria (and polydipsia) is an adverse effect that can occur during treatment initiation and later in treatment secondary to nephrogenic diabetes insipidus. **[Q. p. 199]**

226 **Answer: C.** Narcissistic personality disorder is not described in the ICD-10 classification. Schizotypal disorder is listed under personality disorders in DSM-IV, but with schizophrenia etc. in ICD-10. **[J. pp. 658–1]**

227 **Answer: C.** 'Psychological treatments in schizophrenia: I & II', a meta-analysis of randomised controlled trials, examined this area, looking at four therapies: family therapy, CBT, social skills training and cognitive remediation. Family therapy, in particular single family therapy, had clear preventative effects on the outcomes of psychotic relapse and readmission, in addition to benefits in medication compliance. CBT produced higher rates of 'important improvement' in mental state and demonstrated positive effects on continuous measures of mental state at follow-up. CBT also seems to be associated with low drop-out rates. The second paper from this group looked at social skills training and cognitive remediation. A meta-analysis of randomised controlled trials of social skills training and cognitive remediation showed no clear evidence for any benefits of social skills training on relapse rate, global adjustment, social functioning, quality of life or treatment compliance. Cognitive remediation had no benefit on attention, verbal memory, visual memory, planning, cognitive flexibility or mental state. **[Pilling S, Bebbington P, Kuipers E, Garety P. Psychological treatments in schizophrenia: I & II.** *Psychological Medicine.* **2002; 32: 783–91]**

228 **Answer: D.** Donald Winnicott described the notion of the *transitional object*, which are items that serve as substitutes for the child's mother. Alfred Adler, Freud's pupil and individual psychologist, is known for the inferiority complex, and masculine protest. Carl Rogers is associated with unconditional positive regard and person-centred psychotherapy. Erik Erikson is associated with epigenetic theory and the eight psycho-social stages of development. Carl Jung is associated with the collective unconscious and archetypes. **[AV. pp. 223–39]**

229 A patient with bipolar affective disorder is currently on lithium 1000 mg daily. Recently he has been started on painkillers because of painful joints. What is the most likely risk in this situation?

A. Increased risk of hypothyroidism.

B. Risk of erectile dysfunction.

C. Risk of impaired glucose tolerance.

D. Risk of lithium toxicity.

E. Risk of renal toxicity.

230 A 65-year-old woman suffers a stroke in her left superior temporal gyrus. Which of the following is most likely on examination?

A. Broca's dysphasia.

B. *Donald Duck* speech.

C. Dysarthria.

D. Dysfluent expressive dysphasia.

E. Fluent receptive dysphasia.

231 Which of the following personality disorders is not part of the Cluster B of personality disorders in DSM-IV?

A. Antisocial.

B. Borderline.

C. Histrionic.

D. Narcissistic.

E. Paranoid.

232 A 28-year-old man who lives with his parents is referred to you by his GP. He was noted to have marked loss of interest, and withdrawal from activities over the previous year. There is no past psychiatric history suggestive of psychosis or any evidence of overt psychotic symptoms on mental state examination. What is the most likely ICD-10 diagnosis?

A. Catatonic schizophrenia.

B. Hebephrenic schizophrenia.

C. Paranoid schizophrenia.

D. Residual schizophrenia.

E. Simple schizophrenia.

229 **Answer: D.** The risk of lithium toxicity is increased as lithium levels are increased by analgesics. ACE inhibitors, SSRIs, anti-epileptics, antihypertensives, antipsychotics, calcium channel blockers and diuretics can also increase the level of lithium, leading to increased risk of toxicity. [**AB. p. 328**]

230 **Answer: E.** Broca's dysphasia is secondary to damage in the inferior frontal gyrus and is more properly known as dysfluent expressive dysphasia. Dysarthria is difficulty in the articulation of speech. *Donald Duck* speech (spastic dysarthria) is a sign of pseudobulbar palsy. Fluent receptive dysphasia is also known as Wernicke's dysphasia and is due to damage in the posterior part of the auditory association cortex in the superior temporal gyrus. [**Y. pp. 58–9**]

231 **Answer: E.** Paranoid personality disorder is part of Cluster A, along with schizoid and schizotypal. The other options A–D make up Cluster B. Cluster C includes avoidant, dependent, and obsessive compulsive personality disorders. [**AH. pp. 287–97**]

232 **Answer: E.** In ICD-10 simple schizophrenia is defined as an uncommon disorder with insidious onset, with inability to meet the demands of society. Delusions and hallucinations are not evident. There is marked loss of interest, idleness, and social withdrawal over a period of at least one year. In residual schizophrenia, prominent negative schizophrenic symptoms predominate; however, there should be evidence of one clear-cut psychotic episode. [**I. pp. 89–95**]

233 Which of the following cognitive distortions is not associated with the cognitive theory of depression?

A. Arbitrary inference.   B. Catastrophic thinking.

C. Minimisation.   D. Overgeneralisation.

E. Selective abstraction.

234 Which of the tests below is an objective test of personality?

A. Benton Visual Retention Test.

B. Minnesota Multiphasic Personality Inventory (MMPI).

C. The Rorschach Test.

D. Thematic Appreciation Test (TAT).

E. Wisconsin Card Sorting Test (WCST).

235 The limbic system is thought to be important in the production of the positive symptoms of psychosis. Which of the following structures is not part of this system?

A. Amygdala.   B. Cingulate gyrus.

C. Hippocampal formation.   D. Mammillary bodies.

E. Substantia nigra.

236 Which of the following scenarios best illustrates the defence mechanism of displacement?

A. An overweight woman has been advised to exercise by her GP. She decides not to take exercise as her parents, who were also both overweight, died with cardiac problems and she thinks exercising could put undue pressure on her heart.

B. A man who has been diagnosed with terminal cancer is belligerent with and demanding of medical staff.

C. A man who is dissatisfied with his work accuses his wife of being disappointed in him and his achievements.

D. A woman notices a large hard lump in her breast. She stops her regular breast examination and does not attend her GP.

E. A woman whose mother died recently begins attending church regularly, having not attended church in a number of years. Her mother was a regular church attender.

233 **Answer: B.** Catastrophic thinking is a cognitive distortion found in anxiety disorders. Magnification is another cognitive distortion found in depression along with the ones listed in A, C, D and E. **[H. p. 363]**

234 **Answer: B.** The Minnesota Multiphasic Personality Inventory is an objective test of personality. The Rorschach and Thematic Appreciation Tests are projective tests of personality, as the tests involve the use of ambiguous and unstructured stimuli, e.g. ink blots and pictures. The Benton Visual Retention Test is a test of short-term memory. The Wisconsin Card Sorting Test tests for frontal lobe pathology: it assesses the executive functions of problem solving and abstract reasoning. **[AV. pp. 194–201]**

235 **Answer: E.** Some authors disagree about what makes up the limbic system depending on whether it is defined in terms of its function, development or its connections. **[Y. pp. 98–9]**

236 **Answer: B.** Option B illustrates displacement, the transfer of emotion from a person, object, or situation with which it is properly associated to a lesser source of distress. Option A illustrates rationalisation, the unconscious provision of a false but acceptable explanation for behaviour that has a less acceptable origin. Option C illustrates projection, the attribution to another person of thoughts or feelings similar to one's own thereby rendering one's own thoughts or feelings more tolerable. Option D illustrates denial, when a person behaves as if unaware of something that she may be reasonably expected to know. Option E illustrates identification, the unconscious adoption of the characteristics or activities of another person, often to reduce the pain of separation or loss. **[AG. p. 136]**

237 A 48-year-old male with an ICD-10 diagnosis of alcohol dependence syndrome and alcohol-related liver damage requests disulfiram (Antabuse) to help him stop drinking. What type of conditioning is being used in taking disulfiram?

A. Avoidance.

B. Covert sensitisation.

C. Escape.

D. Punishment.

E. Reward.

238 Choose the most correct statement regarding the Wechsler Adult Intelligence Scale (WAIS).

A. Arithmetic ability is a verbal skill assessment.

B. Digit span is a performance skill test.

C. Five verbal skills are tested.

D. Performance skills are not assessed.

E. Six performance skills are tested.

239 In a school students are awarded with a star for good performance. The star is an example of which of the following?

A. Classical conditioning.

B. Operational conditioning.

C. Primary reinforcement.

D. Pro-social behaviour.

E. Secondary reinforcement.

240 A confused patient is referred to you from the Emergency Department. On examination you note that the patient's left eye is paralysed and fully adducted. Which of the following would you diagnose?

A. 3rd cranial nerve palsy.

B. 4th cranial nerve palsy.

C. 5th cranial nerve palsy.

D. 6th cranial nerve palsy.

E. 7th cranial nerve palsy.

237 **Answer: A.** Punishment is an aversive consequence that suppresses a response, reducing the likelihood of a future response. Avoidance conditioning is where the response prevents an aversive event occurring. Escape conditioning is where the learnt response provides complete escape from the aversive event which remains unchanged. Covert sensitisation is aversive conditioning when performed in the imagination. [**F. p. 3**]

238 **Answer: A.** Arithmetic ability is tested as one of the six (not five) verbal skills in the Wechsler Adult Intelligence Scale (WAIS). There are five performance tests in the WAIS. The digit span is a test of immediate retention and recall; it is a verbal skill test. [**AV. p. 194**]

239 **Answer: E.** This is secondary reinforcement. A primary reinforcement has intrinsic value for the organism, such as water and food. A secondary reinforcer has acquired value for the organism, such as money, medals, diplomas or trophies. The other three options do not apply in this question. [**AC. p. 79**]

240 **Answer: D.** The 7th (facial) and 5th (trigeminal) cranial nerves do not innervate the external muscle of the eyes. The 3rd (oculomotor) nerve serves all the external muscle of the eyes except for the lateral rectus and the superior oblique. Paralysis of the superior oblique muscle causes diplopia on looking down. The 6th cranial nerve is the abducens and causes lateral rectus palsy. [**Y. pp. 153, 156**]

241 A 72-year-old woman is referred for assessment by her GP. He is concerned the she is experiencing abnormal grief following the death of her husband five months previously following a long illness. Which of the following symptoms would suggest that this woman is experiencing an abnormal grief reaction?

A. Guilt.

B. Hallucinations.

C. Panic attacks.

D. Retardation.

E. Sleep disturbance.

242 In explaining to the family of a newly diagnosed patient with schizophrenia the psychological models of the illness, which of the following psychological models is best supported by the evidence?

A. Abnormal communications.

B. Double-bind communications.

C. Expressed emotion.

D. Marital schism.

E. Marital skew.

243 A 29-year-old woman who gave birth one week ago presented with a few days' history of insomnia and irritability, which was followed by confusion, excitability, hallucinations and labile mood. In this condition, all of the following are correct, except:

A. It is commoner among first-time mothers.

B. It has a strong affective component.

C. It is strongly associated with an excess of stressors in the perinatal period.

D. The incidence is 1.5 per 1000 deliveries.

E. There is an association with family psychiatric history.

244 Which of the following is part of the 'four principles' approach to ethics in psychiatry?

A. Beneficence.

B. Maleficence.

C. Non-beneficence.

D. Respect for authority.

E. Unconditional positive regard.

241 **Answer: D.** Many bereaved people experience guilt that they failed to do enough for the deceased. About one in 10 will experience brief hallucinations. Sleep disturbance is very common, and anxiety may occur as panic attacks. An abnormal grief reaction occurs when the symptoms are more intense than usual and meet the criteria for a depressive disorder, if they are prolonged beyond six months, or if they are delayed in onset. This woman demonstrates many of the symptoms of normal grief. However, the symptom of retardation is seldom present in uncomplicated grief, and suggests that she is experiencing abnormally intense grief. **[AG. pp. 152–3]**

242 **Answer: C.** *Marital skew/schism* (Lidz), *abnormal communications* (Wynne and Singer), *double-bind* (Bateson), and *schizophrenogenic mother* (Fromm–Reichmann) are theories that are now disregarded. *Expressed emotion* (Vaughn and Leff) has a good evidence base. **[F. pp. 63–4]**

243 **Answer: C.** This question refers to puerperal psychosis. Its incidence is 1.5 per 1000 deliveries and it is associated with primigravida status. A family history of major psychiatric disorders increases the risk of puerperal psychosis. There has been little evidence of an excess of psychological stresses in the perinatal period. Puerperal psychoses are divided into affective psychoses (70%), schizophrenia (25%) and organic psychoses (the rest). **[H. p. 379]**

244 **Answer: A.** *Beneficence*. The four principal approaches to ethics are: (1) beneficence: the requirement for doctors to do good; (2) nonmaleficence: the requirement to do no harm; (3) justice: ensuring fairness and equity; and (4) respect for autonomy: patients must be accorded the opportunity to make their own decisions, acting as free, autonomous agents. **[A. p. 838]**

245 The extra-pyramidal side-effects (EPSEs) of phenothiazine antipsychotics are caused by which one of the following?

A. Acetylcholine receptor antagonism in the substantia nigra.

B. Acetylcholine receptor antagonism in the striatum.

C. Dopamine receptor agonism in the cortex.

D. Dopamine receptor antagonism in the striatum.

E. Dopamine receptor antagonism in the substantia nigra.

246 Which of the following psychiatric disorders occurs with equal frequency in men and women?

A. Agoraphobia.

B. Generalised anxiety disorder.

C. Panic disorder.

D. Simple phobia.

E. Social phobia.

247 A 26-year-old male newly diagnosed with schizophrenia tells you, as his treating psychiatrist, that he has looked on the Internet for an explanation of the illness. He asks you about the hypotheses listed below. Which of the following hypotheses do you tell him has the best evidence?

A. Continuum.

B. Deficit.

C. Neurodegenerative.

D. Neurodevelopmental.

E. Single aetiological process.

248 With reference to moral philosophies in medicine, which of the following is least correct?

A. Deontology is of Greek origin.

B. Deontology relates to rules, rights and liberty.

C. Teleological morality is also known as utilitarianism.

D. Teleology uses the concept of 'the greatest good for the greatest number'.

E. Teleological morality is concerned with rights rather than the person's interests.

245 **Answer: D.** EPSEs are caused by dopamine receptor blockade in the striatum leading to excess acetylcholine activity. **[Z. p. 39]**

246 **Answer: E.** Social phobia is the only anxiety disorder to occur equally frequently in men and women. The other anxiety disorders occur approximately twice as frequently in women as in men. **[AG. pp. 166–78]**

247 **Answer: D.** The neurodevelopmental model has the most evidence. The continuum model (Crow) postulates a single psychosis with schizophrenia the most severe form, and affective disorders least severe. The neurodegenerative hypothesis has little evidence to support it while the single aetiological process has none. The deficit syndrome (Carpenter) is a specific symptom cluster, with prominent negative symptoms, and is not an aetiological model. **[H. pp. 30–1]**

248 **Answer: E.** Teleology (or utilitarianism) is not concerned with rights of patients (unlike deontology, which deals with rights, obligations and duties). It holds that people (as a group) have interests, instead of rights, and that success or failure in achieving these interests dictates what is right or wrong: actions that suit the most number of interests tend to be the best. **[A. pp. 834–5]**

249 The moon appears larger on the horizon than when it is overhead. This is best explained by which of the following?

A. Accommodation.

B. Binocular vision.

C. Law of effect.

D. Ponzo illusion.

E. Retinal disparity.

250 Which one of the following is an excitatory neurotransmitter?

A. All are inhibitory neurotransmitters.

B. Gamma-amino butyric acid (GABA).

C. Glutamate.

D. Glycine.

E. Serine.

251 A 50-year-old man with schizophrenia is noted on examination to move his arm in response to slight pressure on it, despite being instructed to resist the pressure. Which of the following movement disorders is he exhibiting?

A. Ambitendence.

B. Mannerism.

C. *Mitgehen*.

D. Stereotypy.

E. Waxy flexibility.

252 A 31-year-old woman presents for assessment: her complaint is of sleep disturbance and low mood, secondary to the stressor of a recent divorce. She has no past personal or family psychiatric history. She is finding it difficult to cope with her job. On mental state examination she discloses that she has suicidal ideation. Which of the following would be criteria for admission?

A. A close confiding relationship with her sister.

B. Family living nearby who are willing to take her into their care.

C. Hearing voices while wide awake, alone at home, telling her to kill herself.

D. Reduced self-confidence.

E. Reduced self-esteem.

249 **Answer: D.** Ponzo illusions are the illusions which are associated with linear perspective. All the other answers are distracters here. The law of effect is another name for reinforcement which describes retention of a learned behaviour because of satisfactory results. Binocular vision is simply vision with two eyes, while retinal disparity is the difference in the retinal images caused by the two eyes getting slightly different views of an object. **[AC. p. 64]**

250 **Answer: C.** Glutamate is an excitatory neurotransmitter and acts as an agonist at NMDA, AMPA and Kainate receptors. GABA and glycine are inhibitory neurotransmitters. **[R. p. 229; T. p. 583]**

251 **Answer: C.** Ambitendence occurs when the patient begins to make a movement but, before completing it, starts the opposite movement; for example, bending up and down over a chair without sitting on it. A mannerism is a normal purposeful movement that appears to have social significance but is unusual in appearance. A stereotypy is a repeated purposeless movement. Waxy flexibility occurs when the patient allows himself to be placed in an awkward posture which he then maintains without distress for much longer than most people could achieve without significant discomfort. **[AG. pp. 249–50]**

252 **Answer: C.** Lowered self-esteem and self-confidence, commonly associated with depressive illness, are not in of themselves reason for admission. Good family support and a close confiding relationship are protective. Emergence of psychotic symptoms, in this case a first-episode psychosis, along with increased risk due to command hallucination, are indications for admission. **[AP. p. 244]**

253 You are seeing a 93-year-old man who is on a number of different medications. You are concerned about changes that occur with ageing which may affect his ability to metabolise his medications. Those changes include all the following except:

A. Decreased blood flow in the splanchnic circulation.

B. Decreased proportion of body mass that is composed of muscle.

C. Decreased rate of gastric emptying.

D. Increased gastric pH.

E. Increased proportion of body mass that is composed of water.

254 Which is incorrect regarding the introduction of physical treatments in psychiatry?

A. Iproniazid has antituberculosis effect.

B. Cade is associated with lithium salt.

C. Chlorpromazine was initially used as a sedative.

D. Delay and Deniker are associated with chlorpromazine.

E. None of the above is correct.

255 Which of the following psychiatric disorders has the highest lifetime risk of suicide?

A. Alcohol dependence.

B. Bipolar affective disorder.

C. Major depressive disorder.

D. Opiate dependence.

E. Schizophrenia.

256 An 18-year-old woman is referred for assessment by her GP who reports that she has lost over 20 kg in the past year. The woman admits that she has been restricting her diet as she believes that she is very overweight. She also admits that she self-induces vomiting two or three times per day. She has also begun using laxatives. She goes to the gym daily and twice on Saturday and Sunday. She has not menstruated in the last six months. Which of the following would most likely represent the biochemical profile of this woman?

A. $K^+\downarrow$, amylase $\uparrow$, $Ca^{2+}\downarrow$, phosphate$\downarrow$.

B. $K^+\uparrow$, amylase $\uparrow$, $Ca^{2+}\downarrow$, phosphate$\downarrow$.

C. $K^+\downarrow$, amylase $\downarrow$, $Ca^{2+}\uparrow$, phosphate$\uparrow$.

D. $K^+\uparrow$, amylase $\uparrow$, $Ca^{2+}\uparrow$, phosphate$\uparrow$.

E. $K^+\uparrow$, amylase $\uparrow$, $Ca^{2+}\uparrow$, phosphate$\downarrow$.

253 **Answer: E.** While A to D are true, the proportion of body mass that is comprised of water decreases with age. **[G. p. 398]**

254 **Answer: E.** Iproniazid is an MAOI, and was historically used in tuberculosis treatment. B, C and D are also correct, therefore E is incorrect. **[A. p. 4]**

255 **Answer: B.** For bipolar affective disorder the lifetime risk of death by suicide is 15–20%. The lifetime risk for death by suicide for the remaining options is approximately 10%. **[P. pp. 1184, 2447]**

256 **Answer: A.** This patient has anorexia nervosa, purging type. Patients with anorexia nervosa may become hypokalaemic secondary to vomiting. Amenorrhoea is associated with negative calcium balance with loss of skeletal calcium in the range of 4% per year. Many eating disorder patients have significant bone mineral deficiency, usually osteopenia. Salivary amylase may be increased when purging is present. **[P. pp. 2014–15]**

257 Which of the following is not a common indication for ECT?

  A. Catatonic schizophrenia.
  B. Mania.
  C. Post-ictal psychosis.
  D. Puerperal depressive illness.
  E. Severe depressive illness.

258 Choose the correct option below:

  A. Cerletti and Bini are associated with psychosurgery.
  B. Greisinger believed that mental illnesses are somatic illnesses of the brain.
  C. Kuhn initially introduced clozapine to psychiatry.
  D. Moniz and Sakel advocated insulin coma as a treatment for schizophrenia.
  E. None of the options above is correct.

259 A woman with bipolar affective disorder had three previous episodes of mania and five episodes of depression in the last three years. Her episodes of relapse led to marked psychosocial impairment. Currently she is stable on lithium therapy and wants to become pregnant. What would be the most appropriate advice from the list below that you will offer this woman?

  A. She should be changed to other mood stabilisers such as carbamazepine.
  B. She should be started on another mood stabiliser along with lithium.
  C. She should continue lithium with strict observation and informed consent.
  D. She should discontinue lithium.
  E. She should not get pregnant.

260 A patient is left-handed. Which is the most likely of the following statements?

  A. He has a 70% chance of bilateral (equal) hemisphere dominance for speech.
  B. He has a 70% chance of left hemisphere dominance for speech.
  C. He has a 70% chance of right hemisphere dominance for speech.
  D. He has a 95% chance of right hemisphere dominance for speech.
  E. He will be more artistically gifted.

257 **Answer: C.** A, B, D and E are common indications for ECT. Post-ictal psychosis is not a common indication for ECT. For further reading on post-ictal disorders and twilight states, review Lishman's *Organic Psychiatry*, Chapter 7. **[G. p. 215, L. p. 257]**

258 **Answer: B.** Cerletti and Bini are associated with electroconvulsive treatment. Kuhn is associated with the introduction of the tricyclic anti-depressant imipramine. Sakel was associated with insulin coma treatment but Moniz was associated with psychosurgery. **[A. pp. 4–6]**

259 **Answer: C.** People who have high risk of relapse should preferably con-tinue lithium therapy during pregnancy though with informed consent, appropriate counselling and detailed ultrasound and echocardiography at 16–18 weeks of gestation. Carbamazepine has a higher risk of neural tube defects and should be avoided during pregnancy. **[AB. p. 331]**

260 **Answer: B.** Depending on the assessment method, left-handed patients have an approximately 70% chance of left cerebral hemisphere domi-nance, a 15% chance of right cerebral hemisphere dominance and a 15% chance of equal dominance. **[L. p. 40]**

261 You suspect Huntington's Chorea in a 35-year-old man. Which one of the following findings supports this diagnosis?

A. A mutation on chromosome 14.

B. Greater than 35 repeats of the nucleotide triplet CAT on chromosome 4.

C. Low levels of caeruloplasmin.

D. Normal EEG.

E. Atrophy of the caudate nucleus on MRI scan.

262 A patient under your care was commenced on haloperidol by intra-muscular injection for treatment of severe agitation associated with psychotic symptoms. Seventy-two hours later he developed muscular rigidity, pyrexia and clouding of consciousness. Laboratory results show increased potassium and creatinine phosphokinase. What is the most likely diagnosis in this case?

A. Akathisia.

B. Heat shock.

C. Malignant hyperpyrexia.

D. Neuroleptic malignant syndrome.

E. Tardive dyskinesia.

263 What is the life event below that has the highest life change value according to the Holmes & Rahe Social Readjustment Rating Scale?

A. Being sacked from a job.

B. Death of spouse.

C. Divorce.

D. Jail term.

E. Personal injury or illness.

264 In the nosology of diseases in psychiatry, which option is most correct?

A. As knowledge of specific aetiology improves, diagnostic reliability disimproves.

B. Classification based on treatment response is useful in classification.

C. Classification based on illness outcome is useful in classification.

D. Clinical symptoms in psychiatry include the patient's subjective experiences.

E. Most psychiatric disorders are monothetic.

261 **Answer: E.** Huntington's is caused by a *CAG* tri-nucleotide repeat on chromosome 4. Low levels of caeruloplasmin are found in Wilson's disease. The EEG typically has low amplitude waves. **[L. pp. 466, 470]**

262 **Answer: D.** Neuroleptic malignant syndrome (NMS) is a rare disorder with an incidence of 0.02–2.4%. It has been reported to have 20% mortality. It usually affects young males who are neuroleptic naive. Heat shock and malignant hyperpyrexia are differential diagnoses. Tardive dyskinesia is a syndrome of involuntary movements developing in the course of long-term exposure to antipsychotics. Akathisia is subjective restlessness, associated with an urge to move a part or all of the body. **[A. pp. 93–5; H. pp. 319–20]**

263 **Answer: B.** Death of a spouse is the life event with the highest life change value according to the Holmes & Rahe Social Readjustment Rating Scale with 100 points. The order of the other items is (relative scale points in brackets): divorce (73), jail term (63), personal injury or illness (53) and being sacked from a job (47). **[G. p. 76]**

264 **Answer: D.** Few psychiatric disorders can be said to have one distinctively pathognomonic symptom (monothetic). Most disorders are still defined by a cluster of symptoms (polythetic), some of which may include the patient's subjective experiences. Classification based on treatment response or clinical outcome are both impractical: there are few illness-specific treatments in psychiatry and having to wait to see how the illness turns out in order to diagnose it is not feasible. **[A. pp. 266–7]**

265 Your consultant asks you to prescribe the most serotonergic tricyclic antidepressant for a patient with obsessive compulsive disorder. Which one of the following medications is the best choice?

A. Amitriptyline.

B. Clomipramine.

C. Desipramine.

D. Nortriptyline.

E. Trimipramine.

266 A 28-year-old man with schizophrenia reports that his wife has been replaced by a double. Which of the following syndromes is this man exhibiting?

A. Capgras' syndrome.

B. Couvade syndrome.

C. De Clerambault's syndrome.

D. Fregoli syndrome.

E. Othello syndrome.

267 A 38-year-old woman will not leave her home due to feelings of fear, shortness of breath and palpitations when she does leave home or is in crowds. Which diagnosis is most likely in her case?

A. Agoraphobia.

B. Generalised anxiety disorder.

C. Obsessive compulsive disorder.

D. Panic disorder.

E. Social phobia.

268 Institutionalisation according to Wing and Brown (1970) includes the following, except:

A. Authoritarianism.

B. Depersonalisation.

C. Derealisation.

D. Restriction of independence.

E. Social understimulation.

265 **Answer: B.** Clomipramine is the tricyclic with the most potency for inhibition of serotonin reuptake, whereas desipramine has the most potency for inhibition of noradrenalin reuptake. **[AA. p. 154]**

266 **Answer: A.** In Capgras' syndrome or delusion of doubles the patient believes that a person known to him, usually a close relative, has been replaced by an exact double. In Fregoli syndrome the patient believes that ordinary people in his environment are persecutors in disguise. In De Clerambault's syndrome the patient believes that another person loves him intensely. The object of the delusion is often of higher social status. In Couvade syndrome a person develops extreme anxiety and various physical symptoms of pregnancy when their partner is pregnant. Othello syndrome involves a delusion of infidelity on the part of a sexual partner. **[H. pp. 160–3]**

267 **Answer: A.** This woman is experiencing agoraphobia: it is characterised by avoidance of the phobic situation. This can be from two of the following four: (1) crowds; (2) public places; (3) travelling away from home; and (4) travelling alone. The psychological or autonomic symptoms must be primary manifestations of anxiety and not secondary to other symptoms, i.e. delusions or obsessions. Social phobic or obsessional symptoms if present do not invalidate the diagnosis, so long as they do not dominate the clinical picture. Panic disorder in agoraphobia can be coded in ICD-10 with a fifth character. Generalised anxiety disorder is 'free floating' anxiety and is not restricted to any one environment. **[I. pp. 135–6, 140]**

268 **Answer: C.** Derealisation is not a part of the definition of institutionalisation according to Wing and Brown (1970). All other options in the question are part of the definition in addition to loss of skills. **[H. p. 368]**

269 Which of the following statements is true regarding classification in psychiatry?

   A. All the other options are incorrect.

   B. Categorical approaches to classification are more flexible than dimensional.

   C. Categorical classifications are not often used in psychiatry.

   D. Dimensional approaches to classification are more flexible than categorical.

   E. The classification of psychiatric disorders is generally dimensional.

270 Your consultant asks you to review the long-standing phenothiazine antipsychotic medication that a patient is prescribed for chronic schizophrenia. Following the latest NICE guidelines, which one of the following actions will you take?

   A. Change the prescription to an atypical (second-generation) antipsychotic.

   B. Continue prescribing the phenothiazine.

   C. Discuss the financial implications with the patient.

   D. Let the carer decide.

   E. Review the patient's symptoms, adverse effects and wishes and make a joint decision concerning the antipsychotic.

271 A right-handed 72-year-old man develops right-left disorientation, finger agnosia, dyscalculia, and dysgraphia. Which cerebral lobe is most likely to have been injured?

   A. Left parietal lobe.   **B.** Left temporal lobe.

   C. Right frontal lobe.   **D.** Right parietal lobe.

   E. Right temporal lobe.

272 An 18-month-old child uses its cot blanket to comfort itself in situations that are new. Which of the terms describes this use of the cot blanket?

   A. Capacity to be alone.   **B.** Ejection of the superego.

   C. Idealisation.   **D.** Potential space.

   E. Transitional object.

269 **Answer: D.** Psychiatric classifications have been historically categorical, where disorders are located in mutually exclusive groups, e.g. schizophrenia, affective disorders etc. Dimensional classifications, however, make for greater nosological flexibility and finer distinctions are possible. **[A. pp. 277–8]**

270 **Answer: E.** Financial considerations may come into play if there are two or more second-generation antipsychotics that may be used: the cheaper one should be prescribed in that instance according to NICE. **[V. p. 28]**

271 **Answer: A.** Injury of the posterior parietal lobe can result in Gerstmann's syndrome, characterised by right-left disorientation, finger agnosia (inability to recognise the fingers), dyscalculia (a defect in the ability to use mathematical symbols) and dysgraphia (disorder of writing not related to paralysis of the hands). In a right-handed person this indicates damage to the left parietal lobe. **[H. p. 169; AL. p. 140]**

272 **Answer: E.** A transitional object is an object which is neither oneself nor another person, which is used by an infant for anxiety reduction and self-soothing. Often a blanket or soft toy is used. This object helps in the process of separation and individuation. Capacity to be alone in the presence of another is where the mother allows her child to become increasingly autonomous, while at the same time being dependent on the mother. The potential space is an area of experiencing existing between the baby and the object. All three terms above are described by Winnicott. Idealisation is a Freudian defence mechanism where the object's qualities are elevated to the point of perfection. Ejection of the superego is a Kleinian stage of development during the first year. **[G. pp. 102–4]**

273 With regards to diagnostic classifications, which is correct?

A. Hysteria is an aetiologically important concept in ICD-10.

B. In DSM-IV, Alcohol Misuse is coded on Axis II.

C. In DSM-IV, clinical syndromes on Axis II include Down's syndrome.

D. ICD-10 distinctions between neurosis and psychosis are clearly delineated.

E. Occupational functioning in the last six months is coded on Axis V in DSM-IV.

274 A man has been through severe trauma recently in his life. Which of the following is a protective factor against the development of post-traumatic stress disorder?

A. Lower social class.

B. Being of Afro-Caribbean origin.

C. Low education.

D. Male sex.

E. Previous traumatic events.

275 Choose the most sedating tricyclic antidepressant.

A. Dothiepin.   B. Imipramine.

C. Lofepramine.   D. Nortryptyline.

E. Trimipramine.

276 Which of the following figures best represents the proportion of people with a mental health problem who receive their treatment in a primary care setting?

A. 5%.   B. 10%.

C. 20%.   D. 30%.

E. 50%.

273 **Answer: C.** Developmental syndromes like Down's syndrome can be coded on Axis II of DSM-IV. Hysteria and other terms devoid of significant aetiological significance are expunged from ICD-10. Occupational functioning in the last one year (not six months) is coded on Axis V. **[A. pp. 274–5]**

274 **Answer: D.** Risk factors for the development of PTSD include: low education status, lower social class, female sex, pre-morbid low self-esteem, previous history of psychiatric problems and previous traumatic events. **[AB. pp. 368–9]**

275 **Answer: E.** Trimipramine gives profound sedation. Dothiepin is also sedating whereas nortriptyline, lofepramine and imipramine are less sedating. **[V. p. 222; AI. pp. 47–8]**

276 **Answer: E.** The prevalence of diagnosable mental disorder in the general population is around 20% and more than one half of these people get their psychiatric care from their GP. It is estimated that mental health problems constitute approximately 25% of consultations with GPs. GPs refer only 5–10% of the mental health problems they see on to a psychiatrist. **[P. p. 2228]**

277 A 30-year-old woman presents to you with a phobia of insects. She describes to you that as a young child that she remembers being severely stung by wasps. She now has a fear of wasps along with what she describes as 'all flying and crawling insects'. What term best describes her fear of all such insects?

A. Discrimination.

B. Extinction.

C. Generalisation.

D. Higher-order conditioning.

E. Incubation.

278 Choose the most correct statement in relation to categorical and dimensional classification of diseases.

A. Categorical classifications are more difficult to understand.

B. Categorical classifications can easily be converted into dimensional.

C. Dimensional classifications are more acceptable to psychiatrists.

D. Dimensional classifications can easily be converted to categorical.

E. Personality disorders lend themselves easily to categorical classification.

279 A man with post-traumatic stress disorder wants to discuss with you his long-term prognosis. From the list below, which factor may prevent his recovery?

A. Absence of avoidance.

B. Being ignored by others.

C. No further traumatic events.

D. Normal pre-morbid functioning.

E. Supportive family.

280 You wish to prescribe a very short acting oral benzodiazepine for an osteoporotic elderly patient with generalised anxiety disorder who needs an MRI as an outpatient but is terrified of the scan. Which of the following is the most suitable?

A. Diazepam.

B. Chlordiazepoxide.

C. Flurazepam.

D. Promethazine.

E. Triazolam.

277 **Answer: C.** Generalisation in classical conditioning is where the conditioned response (CR) once established can be transferred to a stimulus that is similar to the conditioned stimulus. **[F. pp. 1–2]**

278 **Answer: D.** An advantage of dimensional classifications is their inherent flexibility. **[A. pp. 277–8]**

279 **Answer: B.** Lack of negative responses from others is a protective factor and helps in recovery. Being ignored or having a negative response from others can prevent complete recovery. All of the other factors listed are good prognostic factors along with good financial situation, no ongoing litigation and no physical disability as a result of trauma. **[AB. pp. 368–9]**

280 **Answer: E.** Triazolam has a $t_{1/2}$ of two to five hours and is without active metabolites and is therefore a suitable choice (midazolam is also short acing but often has a longer duration of amnesia). Diazepam has a long $t_{1/2}$ of up to 100 hours and has active metabolites, as do chlordiazepoxide and flurazepam. It should be noted that a stated $t_{1/2}$ can be prolonged in the elderly. Promethazine is an antihistamine with long-acting sedative qualities. **[Q. p. 181; AA. pp. 42, 117]**

281 A 45-year-old woman with schizophrenia requires a depot antipsychotic. She has been unsuccessfully treated with an atypical depot and a typical depot is being considered. She has a history of third-party auditory hallucinations, persecutory delusions and depressive symptoms when unwell. Which of the following depots would be the most suitable?

A. Flupenthixol decanoate.

B. Fluphenazine decanoate.

C. Haloperidol decanoate.

D. Pipothiazine palmitate.

E. Zuclopenthixol decanoate.

282 A 65-year-old patient with schizophrenia under your care wishes to make a will. Which of the following is not part of testamentary capacity?

A. Ability to challenge jurors.

B. Appreciation of the extent of his assets.

C. Knowledge of the persons who are the objects of the will.

D. Understanding the nature and implications of making a will.

E. Understanding which persons reasonably expect to benefit from the will, and the manner of distributing the assets between them.

283 A 29-year-old woman who gave birth three days ago presented with weeping, feeling depressed and irritable associated with insomnia and poor concentration. In this condition all of the following are correct, except:

A. A biochemical basis is postulated.

B. More common in multigravida.

C. More than 50% of women who give birth may develop it.

D. Premenstrual tension is associated.

E. Weight loss is recognised.

284 Which one of following neuroreceptors is a member of the ligand-gated ion channel 'superfamily' of receptors?

A. Adrenergic.

B. BDNF.

C. $GABA_A$.

D. Muscarinic cholinergic.

E. Serotonergic.

281 **Answer: A.** Flupenthixol decanoate is claimed to be more effective in depressed patients. Zuclopenthixol decanoate is believed to be more effective in aggressive patients, pipothiazine palmitate when EPSEs are problematic, and haloperidol decanoate in the prophylaxis of manic illness. Fluphenazine decanoate is said to be associated with depressed mood. **[V. p. 42]**

282 **Answer: A.** B to D are the requirements for testamentary capacity. Ability to challenge jurors is part of fitness to plead. **[AF. pp. 284, 289–90]**

283 **Answer: B.** This question refers to postpartum blues. All items are correct except B: it is more common among primigravida. **[H. p. 381]**

284 **Answer: C.** GABA$_A$ acts through ligand-gated ion channel receptors, as do glycine, glutamate and nicotinic cholinergic receptors. BDNF (brain-derived neurotrophic factor) receptors are part of the tyrosine kinase-linked receptors superfamily. The G protein-coupled receptors superfamily includes adrenergic, muscarinic cholinergic, and serotonergic receptors. **[A. p. 51]**

285 Tricyclic antidepressants (TCADs) are frequently used to treat depression. Regarding their effects on brain neurochemistry, which of the following statements is most accurate?

A. They decrease central β_1-adrenoceptor density.

B. They decrease the synaptic concentration of both noradrenaline and serotonin.

C. They decrease the synaptic concentration of noradrenaline.

D. They increase central α_2-adrenoceptor density.

E. They inhibit monoamine oxidase.

286 Which of the following figures best represents the proportion of patients who develop agranulocytosis on clozapine treatment?

A. 0. 0001%.

B. 0.1%.

C. 1%.

D. 5%.

E. 10%.

287 A 19-year-old man requests a meeting with you to discuss his possible risk of developing schizophrenia. His father attends your psychiatric service for treatment of a paranoid schizophrenia. Which single item listed below would you advise him to avoid in order to reduce his risk of developing schizophrenia?

A. Alcohol.

B. Cannabis.

C. Cigarettes.

D. High expressed emotion within the family.

E. Stressful employment.

288 Which option is most correct regarding criteria for identification of neurotransmitters?

A. All options below are correct.

B. Postsynaptic concentration control is required.

C. Produced in presynaptic terminal.

D. Released presynaptically by nerve activity.

E. Stored presynaptically in an inactive form.

285 **Answer: A.** Chronic treatment with TCADs leads to down-regulation of central β_1-adrenoceptors and α_2-adrenoceptors. TCADs increase the levels of monoamines by blocking their reuptake. **[AA. p. 157]**

286 **Answer: C.** 0.7% of patients treated with clozapine develop agranulocytosis over one year. Approximately 3% of patients treated with clozapine develop neutropenia. The risk of death from clozapine-induced agranulocytosis is thought to be less than 1/10 000. **[V. pp. 77–8]**

287 **Answer: B.** Cannabis is known to be the most harmful in terms of development of the illness. The Swedish conscript study showed that regular cannabis use (more than 50 times) was associated with an increase risk (odds ratio 6.7) of developing schizophrenia. High expressed emotions at home are more likely to trigger relapse. **[H. p. 74; Zammit S, Allebeck P, Andreasson S, Lundberg I, and Lewis G. Self-reported cannabis use as a risk factor for schizophrenia in Swedish conscripts of 1969: historical cohort study. *BMJ*. 2002; 325: 1199]**

288 **Answer: A.** All the options are required criteria for identification of neurotransmitters. **[A. p. 47]**

289 A 32-year-old woman presents with history of multiple physical complaints for the past four years. These include headaches, abdominal pain, dysmenorrhoea, nausea, food intolerance, and loss of libido. Most recently she has been complaining of difficulty swallowing, and has taken extended sick leave from work. These symptoms have been extensively investigated but no physical cause has been found, although she has been diagnosed with irritable bowel syndrome. What is the most likely diagnosis in this woman's case?

A. Conversion disorder.   B. Hypochondriasis.

C. Major depressive episode.   D. Somatisation disorder.

E. Somatoform pain disorder.

290 A patient who is prescribed chlorpromazine 600 mg per day complains of feeling stiff and you diagnose EPSEs. You decide to change to an equivalent dose of an alternative antipsychotic which is less likely to cause EPSEs. Which of the following will you prescribe?

A. Amisulpride 20 mg per day.

B. Haloperidol 6 mg per day.

C. Quetiapine 400 mg per day.

D. Risperidone 6 g per day.

E. Sulpiride 600 mg per day.

291 Which of the following antipsychotics at average daily dose has the highest monthly cost?

A. Amisulpride 800 mg daily.

B. Aripiprazole 20 mg daily.

C. Haloperidol 10 mg daily.

D. Olanzapine 15 mg daily.

E. Risperidone 6 mg daily.

292 A 37-year-old married mother, with an ICD-10 diagnosis of a moderate depressive disorder attends your psychiatric clinic. Which of the following is the most significant vulnerability factor with regard to her depressive disorder?

A. Employed.

B. Loss of mother before age 15 years.

C. Low self-esteem.

D. Two children under the age of 15 years.

E. Supportive relationship with her spouse.

289 Answer: D. In somatisation disorder the patient experiences persistent recurrent multiple physical symptoms starting in early adult life or earlier. There is usually a long history of inconclusive medical and/or surgical investigations and procedures, and high rates of social and occupational impairment. The DSM-IV criteria require four pain symptoms, two gastro-intestinal symptoms, one sexual symptom, and one pseudoneurological symptom for the diagnosis. Conversion disorder involves symptoms or deficits affecting voluntary motor or sensory function, which cannot be fully explained by a general medical condition. Hypochondriasis is distinguished from somatisation disorder by the patient's preoccupation with the underlying cause rather than symptom relief. Somatoform pain disorder is characterised by persistent severe and distressing pain, at one or more anatomical sites, which is not fully explained by a physical disorder. Patients with major depressive disorder may present with non-specific physical complaints, although these are not predominant in the clinical picture. In all of the above disorders the symptoms are not intentionally produced or feigned, distinguishing them from factitious disorder or malingering. **[AH. pp. 229–36]**

290 Answer: C. Amisulpride probably has less risk of EPSEs and could be tried but the above dose would be too low in terms of equivalence. Haloperidol and sulpiride can both cause EPSEs. Risperidone may not cause EPSEs at low doses. Quetiapine generally does not cause EPSEs. **[Z. p. 81]**

291 Answer: B. The proprietary costs (not including dispensing fees, or the costs attached to a private prescription) of the drugs mentioned are as follows:

Amisulpride 800 mg daily	£122.76	€181.12
Aripiprazole 20 mg daily	£217.78	€321.31
Haloperidol 10 mg daily	£6.30	€8.29
Olanzapine 15 mg daily	£127.69	€188.38
Risperidone 6 mg daily	£101.01	€149.02.

[V. p. 18]

292 Answer: C. Vulnerability factors for depressive illness described by Brown and Birley were: unemployment, three or more children under the age of 15 years at home, lack of a supportive relationship with spouse, loss of the mother before age 11 years. Low self-esteem was described in the initial study and was replicated in further studies by Brown. **[H. p. 54; G. p. 74]**

293 Your community psychiatric nurse (CPN) asks you to see a 26-year-old woman who presented two days ago with superficial self-inflicted lacerations following a minor argument at home. The CPN describes the woman as being a somewhat shallow person with labile mood. She enjoys and exaggerates expression of emotions and appears egocentric, self-indulgent and manipulative. She likes to be at the centre of attention and seeks excitement all the time. The most likely diagnosis is:

A. Dependent personality disorder.

B. Emotionally unstable personality disorder – borderline type.

C. Emotionally unstable personality disorder – impulsive type.

D. Histrionic personality disorder.

E. None of the above.

294 Which of these options are correctly paired?

A. G protein-coupled receptors and glutamate.

B. G protein-coupled receptors and glycine.

C. Ligand-gated ion channel receptors and BDNF.

D. Ligand-gated ion channel receptors and visual pigments.

E. Tyrosine kinase-linked receptors and NGF.

295 Which one of the following statements concerning pharmacokinetics is true?

A. Bioavailability is synonymous with bioequivalence.

B. Dopamine crosses the blood–brain barrier with ease.

C. Potency is synonymous with efficacy.

D. The rate of metabolism of a medication with 'zero-order kinetics' does not depend on the concentration of the medication.

E. The volume of distribution of a medication cannot be greater than the volume of total body water.

296 A 72-year-old woman is referred for assessment by her GP. He reports that her family have complained that she is losing her memory. He suspects that she is demonstrating features of pseudodementia rather than dementia. Which of the following features would suggest that he is right?

A. Apraxia.   B. No diurnal mood variation.

C. Normal sleep/wake cycle.   D. Prominent memory disturbance.

E. Rapid onset.

293 **Answer: D.** This woman most likely has histrionic personality disorder. In emotionally unstable personality disorder – impulsive type, there is emotional instability, lack of control associated with outbursts of violence or threatening behaviour. In emotionally unstable personality disorder – borderline type there is affective instability, outbursts of intense anger leading to violence and chronic feelings of emptiness and boredom. On the other hand, persons with dependent personality disorder allow others to make important life decisions for them and are usually uncomfortable or helpless when alone. **[G. pp. 340–1]**

294 **Answer: E.** NGF (nerve growth factor) receptors are part of the tyrosine kinase-linked receptors superfamily of receptors. **[A. p. 51]**

295 **Answer: D.** Alcohol is an example of a substance that has zero-order kinetics – its elimination can become saturated and so does not vary with increased amounts taken beyond this. **[AA. pp. 27–34]**

296 **Answer: E.** Patients with pseudodementia are more likely to present with rapid onset, distressed affect, fluctuating cognitive deficit, islands of normality, with no dyspraxia or dysphasia, and a past or family history of affective disorder. Patients with dementia are more likely to present with a normal sleep/wake cycle, no diurnal variation in symptoms, gradual onset, prominent memory disturbance and focal features such as apraxia, agnosia and dysphasia. However, there can be significant overlap between dementia and pseudodementia, and patients who develop pseudodementia while depressed have a higher incidence of organic dementia at follow-up. **[S. p. 300]**

297 Which of the following treatments was used to aid remembering past trauma and then to bring about catharsis?

A. Abreaction.

B. Electroconvulsant therapy.

C. Insulin coma therapy.

D. Sleep deprivation therapy.

E. Subcaudate tractotomy.

298 Regarding GABA receptors, which is the most correct option?

A. Benzodiazepines have a specific binding site on $GABA_A$ receptors.

B. $GABA_B$ receptors are pharmacologically identical to $GABA_A$ receptors.

C. The $GABA_A$ is not a ligand-gated channel ion.

D. The $GABA_A$ receptor is an excitatory molecule.

E. The ratio of $GABA_A$ to $GABA_B$ receptors in the CNS is roughly 1:1.

299 A 20-year-old actress has been diagnosed with depression. She is quite worried about the side-effects of weight gain associated with anti-depressant medication. From the list below what would be your choice on the basis of available data?

A. Amitriptyline.

B. Clomipramine.

C. Fluoxetine.

D. Mirtazapine.

E. Sertraline.

300 Regarding cognitive behaviour therapy for depression, which of the following statements is false?

A. It is provided by an active therapist.

B. Many trials comparing it to psychodynamic and interpersonal therapies show similar outcomes.

C. Most benefit comes after session eight.

D. Recently 'mindfulness meditation' has been integrated into CBT.

E. The focus is on the present problems.

297 Answer: A. Abreaction was used in psychoanalysis to relive an experience in order to remove the emotion associated with it, i.e. as a means of inducing catharsis. Insulin coma therapy was introduced by Sakel in the 1930s initially for the treatment of drug addiction but advocated later for its use in schizophrenia. Sleep deprivation is used in mood disorders for several reasons, including augmenting the response to antidepressant medication, or as an antidepressant in treatment resistant depression. Subcaudate tractotomy is a type of psychosurgery which is used for the treatment of intractable depressive illness **[A. p. 6; G. p. 216; Mahli, GS, Bartlett JR. Depression: a role for neurosurgery?** *Br J Neurosurg.* **2000; 14: 415–22; Jackson SW. Catharsis and abreaction in the history of psychological healing.** *Psychiatr Clin North Am.* **1994; 17: 471–91]**

298 Answer: A. There is a specific benzodiazepine binding site on $GABA_A$ receptors, which is a ligand-gated channel ion receptor, pharmacologically distinct from $GABA_B$. The $GABA_A$ receptor is inhibitory by nature. $GABA_A$ receptors are more widely distributed in the CNS. **[A. pp. 55–8]**

299 Answer: C. Fluoxetine is associated with weight loss as well as paroxetine and fluvoxamine. Sertraline has been reported to cause limited weight gain while citalopram has no effect on weight. Tricyclic antidepressants are associated with weight gain. Mirtazapine is associated with weight gain also. **[AB. p. 853]**

300 Answer: C. CBT is provided by an active therapist and is present-focused. Most benefit occurs within the first eight sessions, throwing into question the concept of standard 12–16 sessions. Although there is more high-quality research supporting CBT, many studies do not show a sustained difference between the therapies. Mindfulness CBT is a developing area. **[Whitfield G, Williams C. The evidence base for cognitive–behavioural therapy in depression: delivery in busy clinical settings.** *Advances in Psychiatric Treatment.* **2003; 9: 21–30]**

301 A patient with schizophrenia has been started on an atypical antipsychotic. He is complaining of weight gain. From the proposed mechanisms given below, which one is unlikely to cause this side-effect?

A. Activation of 5-HT_{2C} receptors.

B. Altered insulin secretion.

C. Fluid retention.

D. Reduced metabolism.

E. Sedation leading to reduced activity.

302 A 26-year-old male from South East Asia is referred to you with the following symptoms: intense anxiety and a belief that his penis is shrinking into his abdomen. Which of the syndromes below best describes this clinical picture?

A. Amok.   B. Dhat.

C. Pikbloto.   D. Latah.

E. Koro.

303 Which of the following conditions is associated with increased REM (rapid eye movement) sleep?

A. Alcoholism.   B. Anxiety disorder.

C. Benzodiazepine use.   D. Panic disorder.

E. Schizophrenia.

304 A hospital pharmacist has been reviewing some prescriptions for antidepressants made in the service for depressed patients. All of these patients are adults in their thirties and are otherwise healthy. Which of the following does she suspect is an insufficient dose?

A. Amitriptyline 125 mg/day.   B. Duloxetine 60 mg/day.

C. Fluvoxamine 25 mg/day.   D. Lofepramine 140 mg/day.

E. Sertraline 50 mg/day.

301 **Answer: A.** 5-HT$_{2C}$ blockade is responsible for weight gain rather than activation. **[AB. p. 852]**

302 **Answer: E.** Koro is described in males from South East Asia and China, but has been described in other cultures. It involves a period of anxiety along with a belief that the patient's penis is shrinking. When the penis disappears completely the person believes that he will die. Amok is described in Malays where, following a period of withdrawal, the sufferer becomes violent and may kill other people until overcome. If the person survives the period of violence, they pass into a deep sleep with subsequent amnesia for the event. Dhat is common in India, where vague somatic symptoms are sometimes accompanied by sexual dysfunction, and a belief that semen is being lost in the urine, through excessive masturbation, or sexual intercourse. Latah usually occurs in Malay women; it is comprised of an exaggerated startle, coprolalia, echolalia, echopraxia and automatic obedience. Pikbloto is seen in Eskimo women where they take off their clothes which endangers them to cold exposure and run about wildly. It is associated with either suicidal or homicidal behaviour. **[G. pp. 386–8]**

303 **Answer: A.** Alcoholism is associated with increased delta, REM sleep and alpha activity. Panic disorder and anxiety disorders are not associated with REM changes. Schizophrenia is associated with reduced slow-wave sleep and reduced REM sleep. In benzodiazepine use there is reduction in REM and slow-wave sleep with an increase in stage 2 sleep. **[H. p. 207]**

304 **Answer: C.** Fluvoxamine is one of the lesser prescribed SSRIs, possibly because of its propensity to cause nausea. Its minimum effective dose is 50 mg/day and is licensed for doses between 100 and 300 mg/day. Tricyclic antidepressants have unclear minimum effective doses but are thought to require at least 75–125 mg/day. **[V. pp. 180–9]**

305 You are asked to review a 25-year-old patient who has taken an overdose of benzodiazepines. On examination the patient opens his eyes in response to voice, localises to painful stimuli and utters inappropriate words. The correct Glasgow Coma Score is

A. 3   B. 7.

C. 11   D. 13.

E. 15.

306 A 17-year-old male patient with a two-year history of anorexia nervosa is referred for inpatient treatment. Which of the following factors in his history will most worsen his prognosis?

A. Age of onset.   B. Being male.

C. Comorbid depression.   D. Duration of illness.

E. Pre-morbid sexual activity.

307 Lithium bromide and lithium chloride salts have been in use for medicinal purposes since the last century. Which of the following conditions was it used for before its use in psychiatry?

A. Used for the treatment of affective disorders.

B. Used for the treatment of gout.

C. Used for the treatment of hypertension.

D. Used for the treatment of insomnia.

E. Used for the treatment of syphilis.

308 You are discussing pharmacological treatment options for a patient with first onset of schizophrenia. He is worried about developing diabetes as he has read on the Internet that antipsychotics can cause this and he has a maternal aunt who has type II diabetes. Given this, with which of the following agents might you be most able to reassure his fears?

A. Amisulpride.   B. Chlorpromazine.

C. Clozapine.   D. Olanzapine.

E. Quetiapine.

305 **Answer: C.** The Glasgow Coma Scale is scored as follows:

Eyes: Opens eyes spontaneously = 4 / Opens eyes in response to voice = 3 / Opens eyes in response to painful stimuli = 2 / Does not open eyes = 1.
Verbal: Converses normally = 5 / Confused = 4 / Utters inappropriate words = 3 / Incomprehensible sounds = 2 / Makes no sounds = 1.
Motor: Obeys commands = 6 / Localises painful stimuli = 5 / Withdraws from painful stimuli = 4 / Decorticate posturing upon painful stimuli = 3 / Decerebrate posturing upon painful stimuli = 2 / Makes no movements = 1. **[L. p. 167]**

306 **Answer: C.** Bad prognostic signs include psychiatric comorbidity, very young or older age at onset and longer duration of illness. Good prognostic signs in anorexia nervosa are a short duration of illness with onset in the early to mid-teens. There is some controversy whether maleness by itself confers a greater risk of a poor outcome: most texts list this as associated with poor prognosis. However, men with some degree of sexual fantasy or activity before the development of anorexia nervosa have a better outcome. **[P. p. 2017]**

307 **Answer: B.** It was first used in the 1840s for the treatment of gout. Subsequent uses were as a hypnotic and antihypertensive. It was used for the treatment of depressive illness before its anti-manic effects were discovered. **[A. pp. 119–20]**

308 **Answer: A.** Schizophrenia had been associated with impaired glucose tolerance and diabetes even in the pre-antipsychotic era; however, there have been reports of certain antipsychotics being more associated with such problems. Amisulpride appears to offer the least risk among the options offered, although there has been less research done. Among typical antipsychotics, aliphatic phenothiazines have been most implicated. Clozapine and olanzapine are the atypical agents that have been most associated with hyperglycaemia-related problems. Quetiapine has less of an effect than clozapine or olanzapine in this regard but is more associated with diabetes than the typical antipsychotics. **[V. pp. 123–5]**

309 A 17-year-old girl has been brought to your outpatient clinic by her mother after some weight loss. You suspect anorexia nervosa. From the list below which information least supports your diagnosis?

A. She has recently joined the gym.

B. She is worried about putting on weight.

C. She complains of lethargy.

D. Her menstrual cycles have stopped.

E. Her BMI is 17.

310 Which of the following has been discredited as an explanation of the development of delusional thinking?

A. A 'jumping to conclusions' thinking style.

B. Delusional atmosphere.

C. Schizophrenogenic mother.

D. *Sensitiver Beziehungswahn*.

E. Social attribution theory.

311 Which of the following names is most strongly associated with operant conditioning theory?

A. Bandura.

B. Pavlov.

C. Skinner.

D. Thorndike.

E. Watson.

312 A 39-year-old male with a 20-year history of alcohol dependence syndrome with no period of abstinence is referred to you by his GP. He complains of memory loss for events over the past few years and an inability to form new memories. On examination his consciousness is clear and he has peripheral neuropathy. The most likely diagnosis in this man is?

A. Alcohol dementia.

B. Confabulation.

C. Delirium tremens.

D. Korsakoff's syndrome.

E. Wernicke's encephalopathy.

309 **Answer: C.** Patients with anorexia nervosa usually do not complain of lethargy, rather they are overactive and do excessive exercises and use appetite suppressants. All the other options are diagnostic criteria according to ICD-10. **[AB. p. 853]**

310 **Answer: C.** The schizophrenogenic mother was supposed to cause schizophrenia in her offspring by sending mixed messages to her child. **[D. pp. 113–14; T. p. 102]**

311 **Answer: C.** Skinner's ideas of radical behaviourism made the effects of the environment a central feature of learning. Operant conditioning is a form of learning in which behavioural frequency is altered through the application of positive and negative consequences. Thorndike preceded Skinner in identifying the relationship between appropriate behaviour and experiences of success and failure. Pavlov and Watson are associated with classical conditioning, the association of a neutral stimulus with an unconditioned stimulus such that the neutral stimulus comes to bring about a response similar to that originally elicited by the unconditioned stimulus. Pavlov performed experiments examining the idea that learning occurs when two events occur closely together. Watson demonstrated classical conditioning can give rise to phobia-like behaviour in a famous experiment involving an 11-month-old infant in which he paired a loud noise with the sight of a white rat, leading the child to fear the rat and also similar objects, an example of stimulus generalisation. Bandura advocated social cognitive learning theory, which argues that the influence of environmental events on the acquisition and the regulation of behaviour is primarily a function of cognitive processes. **[E. pp. 417–20]**

312 **Answer: D.** Korsakoff's syndrome is the most likely diagnosis in this case. It consists of an inability to form new memories and retrograde amnesia, along with peripheral neuropathy and relative preservation of intellectual function with clear consciousness. Confabulation is also a symptom: this is the apparent recollection of imaginary events and experiences. Wernicke's encephalopathy consists of confusion and clouding of consciousness, nystagmus and ophthalmoplegia. Ataxic gait and peripheral neuropathy are also features. Alcohol dementia rarely occurs before the age of 40 years. In this case it is a differential for Korsakoff's syndrome, but is not the best fit for the clinical picture. **[H. p. 125]**

313 In a 75-year-old man with Alzheimer's dementia, which of the following neuropathological findings is less likely to be present?

- **A.** Balloon cells.
- **B.** Granulovascular degeneration.
- **C.** Hirano inclusion bodies.
- **D.** Neurofibrillary tangles.
- **E.** Senile plaques.

314 A patient with mild depression comes to you looking to be commenced on St John's wort (*Hypericum perforatum*). She says she has researched it on the Internet and bombards you with a number of 'facts'. With which of the following would you most disagree?

- **A.** 'Drop-out rates in trials were less than with SSRIs.'
- **B.** 'It affects both serotonin and noradrenaline.'
- **C.** 'It is not associated with induction of hypomania in bipolar disorder.'
- **D.** 'It is of benefit in mild depression.'
- **E.** 'There is evidence that severely depressed patients may benefit from it.'

315 A 65-year-old woman believes that a male nurse on the ward is her husband. Which delusional misidentification syndrome is this?

- **A.** Capgras.
- **B.** Cotard.
- **C.** Fregoli.
- **D.** Intermetamorphosis.
- **E.** Subjective doubles.

316 A 32-year-old man presents following a road traffic accident 6 months previously in which he was severely injured. He experiences recurrent nightmares of the event, and distressing intrusive memories. He does not drive and avoids the area in which the accident occurred. He will not speak about the accident. What form of learning is thought to contribute to the avoidance symptoms exhibited by this patient?

- **A.** Classical conditioning.
- **B.** Instrumental learning.
- **C.** Modelling.
- **D.** Operant conditioning.
- **E.** Social-cognitive learning.

313 **Answer: A.** Balloon cells are swollen cells with silver-staining inclusion bodies (also called Pick's cells) which are likely to be present in Pick's disease and not Alzheimer's dementia. All of the other options are present in Alzheimer's dementia. **[H. p. 175]**

314 **Answer: C.** You might take issue with most of the statements, citing a relative lack of research, short duration of trials and uncertainty regarding active ingredients and dosage standardisation. Despite this, there is some evidence for each of the statements except that stating that it does not induce hypomania: this has been reported. It has been shown to be of benefit in mild to moderate depression, but there is some evidence that it may be of benefit in severe depression. It is not licensed for treatment of depression in the UK or Ireland. **[V. pp. 244–5]**

315 **Answer: C.** In Cotard's delusion the patient may believe that she has died or does not exist or that parts of the body are missing and so may be part of the spectrum of misidentification syndromes. **[D. p. 118]**

316 **Answer: A.** Classical conditioning explains how stimuli associated with a severe trauma come to elicit stress responses that were part of the original trauma. Instrumental learning is another term for operant conditioning. Modelling is observational learning. Social cognitive theory espouses that the influence of environmental events on the acquisition and the regulation of behaviour is primarily a function of cognitive processes. **[E. pp. 415–20]**

317 In terminally ill people near death, it is believed that the individual passes through several stages. Which of the following is not a stage associated with impending death?

A. Acceptance.

B. Alarm.

C. Anger.

D. Bargaining.

E. Denial.

318 A 24-year-old man has developed epilepsy. Which of the following agents would you consider potentially most harmful to the treatment of his epilepsy?

A. Amitriptyline.

B. Citalopram.

C. Haloperidol.

D. Lithium.

E. Sulpiride.

319 A mother of an anorexic patient wants to discuss prognosis. From the list below what is a good prognostic factor for anorexia nervosa?

A. Anxiety while eating with others.

B. Bulimic features.

C. Female sex.

D. Early age of onset.

E. Rapid weight loss.

320 Which of the following is not one of Schneider's first-rank symptoms of schizophrenia?

A. Auditory hallucinations in 'running commentary' format.

B. Delusional perception.

C. Persecutory delusion.

D. Somatic passivity.

E. Thought insertion.

317 **Answer: B.** In 1969 Kübler-Ross described the following five stages in patients who were terminally ill under her care: shock and denial, anger, bargaining, depression, and acceptance. Alarm is one of the five stages of bereavement. **[G. p. 45]**

318 **Answer: A.** Among antipsychotics, those with low potency and high sedation are most associated with lowering seizure threshold: clozapine is the worst culprit. Lithium is more associated with convulsive effects in overdose. SSRIs have lower potential to cause seizures than other antidepressants, particularly at lower doses. **[V. pp. 354–5]**

319 **Answer: D.** Generally, most texts suggest female sex has a better prognosis than male sex in anorexia nervosa. Other poor prognostic factors are poor parental relationship, poor childhood social adjustment and chronic illness. **[AB. p. 383]**

320 **Answer: C.** Persecutory delusions may be an ICD-10 criterion but unless they are a delusional perception they are not first-rank symptoms. **[T. p. 243]**

321 A 20-year-old woman experiences episodes in which she falls down with a sudden loss of muscle tone after which she sleeps. These episodes tend to be provoked by strong emotion. What symptom is this woman experiencing?

A. Catalepsy.
B. Cataplexy.
C. Catatonia.
D. Cathexis.
E. Sleep paralysis.

322 A 23-year-old female dental hygienist recently treated for a first psychotic episode is reluctant to inform her employer of her illness. She believes that comments her employer had previously made about mentally ill people being dangerous will cause her difficulty in returning to work. Which of the factors below are not likely to increase the prejudice of stigmatisers?

A. Female gender.
B. Homelessness.
C. Perceived course.
D. Perceived danger.
E. Unkempt appearance.

323 A 65-year-old woman presents with more than six months' history of low mood and memory difficulties. Which of the following favours the diagnosis of pseudodementia?

A. A history of depression.
B. Confabulation.
C. Dysphasia.
D. EEG abnormalities.
E. Perseveration.

324 In the diagnosis of ICD-10 Panic Disorder, the following are true except:

A. Choking symptoms are common.
B. If criteria are also met for depressive disorder, panic disorder should not be the main diagnosis.
C. Secondary fears of dying/losing control/going mad are almost invariable.
D. There is no anxiety between attacks.
E. While most attacks last minutes some are longer.

321 **Answer: B.** Cataplexy is temporary sudden loss of muscle tone, causing weakness and immobilisation. It can be precipitated by a variety of emotional states and is often followed by sleep. It is commonly seen in narcolepsy. Catalepsy is a condition in which a person maintains the body position into which they are placed. It is seen in catatonic schizophrenia and is also called waxy flexibility. Cathexis is a term from psychoanalysis meaning a conscious or unconscious investment of psychic energy into an idea, concept, object or person. Sleep paralysis is an episode of inability to move occurring between wakefulness and sleep, in either direction. Catatonic stupor is a state of decreased reactivity to stimuli in which the patient is aware of their surroundings. **[P. pp. 849–59; D. p. 43]**

322 **Answer: A.** Male gender is a more common factor which influences the prejudice of stigmatisers. The following list is from Peter Byrne's article on the 'stigma of mental illness and ways of diminishing it'. The following are likely to increase prejudice: (1) Appearance: unkempt appearance; (2) Behaviour: acute illness episode; (3) Financial circumstances: homelessness; (4) Perceived focus of illness: many deficits; (5) Perceived responsibility: not responsible for actions; (6) Perceived severity: history of hospital admission; (7) Knowledge base about particular disorder: perceived origin: self-inflicted; (8) Perceived course: incurable/'chronic'; (9) Perceived treatments: 'needs drugs' to stay well; (10) Perceived danger: criminality or violence. **[Byrne P. Stigma of mental illness and ways of diminishing it.** *Advances in Psychiatric Treatment.* **2000; 6: 65–72]**

323 **Answer: A.** Features that discriminate dementia from depression or pseudodementia include items B to E, as does sulcal widening on CT. **[H. pp. 171–2]**

324 **Answer: D.** All the statements are contained within the ICD-10 criteria for panic disorder (F41.0) except D. There is *comparative* freedom from anxiety between attacks but the criteria note that anticipatory anxiety is common. **[I. pp. 139–40]**

325 Which one of the following statements concerning the use of language by patients with schizophrenic thought disorder is false?

A. Paragrammatism is when speech is composed of clauses which are individually coherent but which make no sense together in achieving the goal of thought.

B. Paralogia is synonymous with positive thought disorder.

C. The speech is less predictable than normal speech.

D. They have a high type-token ratio.

E. They use stock words.

326 An inpatient with schizoaffective disorder says the following: 'The man in the van, can, can. He has a plan to stand, understand. The band fanned me.' What form of language disorder is he exhibiting?

A. Clang association. B. Echopraxia.

C. Metonymy. D. Palilalia.

E. Verbigeration.

327 Which of the following eminent psychiatrists was first to use the term *schizophrenia*?

A. Bleuler. B. Greisinger.

C. Kahlbaum. D. Kraepelin.

E. Schneider.

328 In the diagnosis of ICD-10 Schizoaffective Disorder, the following statements are false except:

A. A schizoaffective episode invalidates the diagnosis of bipolar affective disorder.

B. Affective and schizophrenic symptoms are prominent and occur within a few days of each other.

C. Florid psychoses are uncommon in schizoaffective disorder, manic type.

D. Mood incongruent delusions in affective disorders suggest schizoaffective disorder.

E. The majority of patients with a schizoaffective disorder, depressive type episode, never recover completely.

325 **Answer: D.** Type-token ratio refers to the number of different words used compared to the number of total words. It has been found to be lower in schizophrenic speech. **[D. pp. 167–9]**

326 **Answer: A.** A clang association is the association of speech directed by the sound of a word rather than by its meaning. It includes punning and rhyming speech and is most often seen in schizophrenia and mania. It has been suggested that the clang associations in the language disorder of schizophrenia involves the initial syllable of a previous word, while the clang in manic speech occurs in terminal syllables. Echolalia is the repeating of words or phrases of one person by another. It is particularly seen in catatonic schizophrenia. Metonymy involves the use of a word or phrase that is related to the proper one but not the one ordinarily used; for example, the patient says he will eat a menu rather than a meal. Palilalia is the repetition of a work or phrase. It is a perseveration phenomenon. Verbigeration is the meaningless and stereotyped repetition of words or phrases seen in schizophrenia. **[P. pp. 849–59; D. p. 167]**

327 **Answer: A.** Eugen Bleuler in 1911 published *Dementia Praecox or the group of Schizophrenias*, and it is his term rather that Kraepelin's *dementia praecox* that became the one universally accepted. Hecker described hebephrenia. Kurt Schneider described first-rank symptoms. **[A. p. 369]**

328 **Answer: B.** Symptoms of both affective and schizophrenic type are prominent and need to occur simultaneously or at least within a few days of each other. Mood-incongruence of psychotic symptoms in otherwise affective disorders is not sufficient for schizoaffective disorder to be diagnosed. Equally, an occasional schizoaffective episode in an otherwise affective disorder does not invalidate the original diagnosis. Florid psychoses are common in manic type but not in depressive type schizoaffective episodes. The majority of patients recover completely from a schizoaffective disorder, depressive type episode, but the prognosis is not as good as for manic type episodes. **[I. pp. 105–8]**

329 A 21-year-old girl presents with symptoms of weight loss and you suspect anorexia nervosa. You want to calculate her Body Mass Index (BMI). Which is the correct formula to calculate BMI?

A. Weight in kilograms divided by height in centimetres squared.

B. Weight in kilograms divided by height in metres squared.

C. Weight in kilograms squared divided by height in metres squared.

D. Weight in kilograms multiplied by 704.5 divided by height in inches squared.

E. Weight in pounds divided by height in metres squared.

330 There are multiple categorisations of schizophrenic thought disorder. Which one of the following associations between clinician and categorisation is incorrect?

A. E. Bleuler – loosening of associations.

B. N. Cameron – defect of deductive reasoning.

C. K. Goldstein – concrete thinking.

D. E. Kraepelin – acataphasia.

E. C. Schneider – derailment.

331 Which of the following brain structures is not included in the limbic system?

A. Amygdala.

B. Hippocampal formation.

C. Hypothalamus.

D. Parahippocampal cingulate gyrus.

E. Posterior nucleus of the thalamus.

332 A 22-year-old woman who lives with her parents presents to you for assessment following the break-up of a short-term relationship. Her parents are concerned that she has expressed suicidal ideation, and has superficially lacerated her left forearm. The most likely diagnosis in this case is:

A. Anankastic personality disorder.

B. Dependent personality disorder.

C. Emotionally unstable personality disorder – borderline type.

D. Emotionally unstable personality disorder – impulsive type.

E. Histrionic personality disorder.

329 **Answer: B.** The BMI is a ratio between weight and height and is a helpful measure to check the risk related to unhealthy weight and body fat. It is a better indicator of predicting health risk compared to body weight alone. **[AB. p. 377]**

330 **Answer: B.** Cameron is associated with asyndesis, which is an inability to preserve conceptual boundaries. **[D. p. 164]**

331 **Answer: E.** The limbic system includes the anterior nucleus of the thalamus. Different authorities list different components, but generally the limbic system includes the hippocampus, mammillary bodies, hypothalamus, anterior nucleus of the thalamus, septal nuclei, fornix, cingulated gyrus, parahippocampal gyrus, amygdala, nucleus accumbens and the mamillothalamic tract. **[S. p. 24]**

332 **Answer: C.** The brief history given points to emotionally unstable personality disorder. The decision as to whether it is impulsive or borderline type is helped by the history of a short-term often 'intense' relationship, along with the episode of deliberate self-harm, in this case pointing to borderline personality type. Impulsive type is characterised by emotional instability and lack of impulse control. Histrionic personality disorder involves shallow and labile affect, suggestibility, self-dramatization, inappropriate seductiveness and over-concern with physical attractiveness. Anankastic and dependent personality disorders can be quickly outruled with the above history. **[I. p. 204]**

333 A 29-year-old woman who presented two weeks after giving birth complained of tearfulness and irritability associated with feeling tired, anxious and worrying about her ability to cope with her baby. She also reported poor appetite, decreased libido and difficulty sleeping. In this condition, all of the following are correct, except:

A. 10% of women develop this in the postpartum period.

B. Aetiological factors include a postulated hormonal effect.

C. It is associated with increased age.

D. It is associated with physical problems in the pregnancy.

E. Most of the cases last more than two months.

334 The general physician has referred a 34-year-old man who has been investigated intensively for years in the general hospital with a variety of symptoms. He suspects hypochondriasis. Which of the following statements from the referral letter is least in keeping with this diagnosis?

A. 'Despite intensive cardiology investigations, the patient still believes he has a serious heart defect.'

B. 'He agrees that referral to a psychiatrist will likely be of benefit.'

C. 'He remains preoccupied with a perceived redness in his cheeks.'

D. 'Several second opinions have been obtained, but the patient has also refused to accept these reassurances.'

E. 'The patient appears depressed.'

335 Andreasen found that several types of thought disorder were characteristic of schizophrenia. Which of the following is not one?

A. Derailment.   B. Illogicality.

C. Neologisms.   D. Loss of goal.

E. Tangentiality.

336 Which of the following patients carries the most risk factors for tardive dyskinesia?

A. A male patient with schizophrenia who has never taken antipsychotic medication.

B. A young female patient with bipolar affective disorder.

C. An elderly female patient with bipolar affective disorder.

D. An elderly female patient with schizophrenia.

E. An elderly male patient with schizoaffective disorder.

333 **Answer: E.** This question refers to puerperal depression: almost 90% last less than one month even without treatment. **[H. p. 381]**

334 **Answer: B.** Patients with hypochondriacal disorder often will not be happy with the referral to a psychiatrist, believing that the physicians/surgeons have 'given up'. Persistent preoccupation with physical appearance can be a presenting symptom. Both persistent belief in at least one serious physical illness despite repeated investigations and repeated refusal to accept reassurance of several doctors are required for definite diagnosis. Depressive and anxiety symptoms are common: comorbid diagnoses can be made if severe enough. **[I. pp. 164–7]**

335 **Answer: C.** Nancy Andreasen found that derailment, illogicality, loss of goal, poverty of speech (poverty of thought), empty speech, alogia, verbigeration and negative formal thought disorder were characteristic of schizophrenia. She found that neologisms and blocking occurred too infrequently to be of diagnostic significance. **[D. p. 164]**

336 **Answer: C.** Although tardive dyskinesia can occur in patients who have never taken antipsychotics, it is much more common in those who have taken antipsychotic drugs for many years. Tardive dyskinesia is more common among women, the elderly and those with diffuse brain pathology. A diagnosis of an affective disorder is also a risk factor. **[H. p. 316]**

337 A 32-year-old man is assessed by you the duty psychiatrist in the A&E department. He has no injuries, and has been cleared by the A&E doctor for psychiatric review of what appear to be psychotic symptoms. Which of the following causes of organic psychosis can be outruled?

A. Alcohol abuse.

B. Amphetamines.

C. Cocaine.

D. Head injury.

E. Hallucinogens.

338 A 42-year-old woman has been referred to your outpatient clinic with suspected alcohol dependence. Using ICD-10 criteria, which of the following is least in keeping with this diagnosis?

A. Her drinking has had little impact on her alternative interests.

B. It takes two bottles of wine for her to become intoxicated.

C. She has been drinking increasing amounts daily for the last five years.

D. She has not experienced any withdrawal state symptoms.

E. She tries to limit her intake but always fails.

339 James, a 70-year-old man, has insomnia and wants sleeping tablets. After seeing him in your OPD you start thinking about the effects of ageing on sleep. From the items given below select the most correct statement about sleep patterns in old age.

A. REM remains stable in old age.

B. REM sleep decreases with age.

C. REM sleep increases with age.

D. The total sleep time increases with age.

E. Total sleep time remains stable with age.

340 The thought disorder found in schizophrenia characterised by monotonous repetition of syllables and words is known as?

A. Echolalia.

B. Logorrhoea.

C. Paraphasia.

D. Verbigeration.

E. Word salad.

337 **Answer: D.** Head injury can be outruled as he has been medically cleared. A detailed drug history and drug screen will identify substance abuse as a potential cause of organic psychosis. **[G. p. 220]**

338 **Answer: A.** She displays diagnostic criteria such as compulsion to drink and tolerance. There appear to be two negatives: lack of withdrawal symptoms and lack of neglect of alternative interests. The lack of withdrawal symptoms is probably explained by lack of abstinence as stated in C. Therefore the lack of impact on alternative interests is the feature least in keeping with alcohol dependence syndrome (F10.2). **[I. pp. 75–7]**

339 **Answer: A.** REM sleep remains stable with age, while the sleep time reduces with increasing age. REM sleep occupies about 20–25% of total sleep time in all ages. **[AB. p. 388]**

340 **Answer: D.** Echolalia is the repetition of words or part of clauses spoken by others. Logorrhoea means verbosity. Paraphasia is a destruction of words with interpolation of garbled sounds. It is also used as a synonym for 'approximate answers'. Word salad is a severe thought disorder where there is a loss of grammatical and syntactical coherence. **[D. pp. 163, 165; M. pp. 63–4]**

341 For which of the following antipsychotic side-effects are anticholinergic drugs unsuitable?

A. Akathisia.
B. Dystonia.
C. Rigidity.
D. Tardive dyskinesia.
E. Tremor.

342 A 30-year-old woman who fears that she has multiple sclerosis was assessed by two physicians for a neurological cause of pain in both her lower limbs and torso. Investigations revealed no neurological cause for the pain. Which is the most likely diagnosis in this case?

A. Anxiety disorder.
B. Depressive disorder.
C. Hypochondriacal disorder.
D. Malingering.
E. Somatisation disorder.

343 A 25-year-old Malaysian woman presents with echolalia, automatic obedience and a hysterical reaction to losing her job. The most likely diagnosis is:

A. Amok.
B. Dhat.
C. Koro.
D. Latah.
E. Susto.

344 Which of the following statements from patients is least likely to indicate a first-rank symptom of schizophrenia?

A. 'Al-Qaeda has implanted a microchip in my skull that makes me think about potential targets for them. The microchip then transmits these thoughts via radio waves to Tora Bora.'

B. 'George W. Bush has replaced my brain with a telegenomic interphrastic pseudocellular organ and derives a malicious pleasure from having done so.'

C. 'I saw Michael Phelps the Olympian hold up his eight gold medals on TV and in that moment I realised I was to swim the Atlantic in order to restore American and European geopolitical relations.'

D. 'My next-door neighbour is abusing me by causing me to have all of his sadness and rage while he steals all of my happiness and pleasure.'

E. 'The voices of the Queen and the Pope discuss me constantly: the Queen demands that I should be executed but the Pope believes I should be saved.'

341 **Answer: D.** The appropriate treatment for tardive dyskinesia is slow withdrawal of or reduction in antipsychotic medication and consideration of an alternative. Anticholinergic medications can provoke or exacerbate tardive dyskinesia. Anticholinergics are an appropriate treatment option for antipsychotic-induced tremor, dystonia and rigidity. Anticholinergics may have some efficacy in treating akathisia which is part of an extra-pyramidal side-effect profile. **[X. pp. 97–104]**

342 **Answer: C.** In this case it is important to distinguish between a somatisation disorder and hypochondriacal disorder. Hypochondriacal disorder is the best answer in this case, as there is a belief in the presence of one physical serious illness underlying the presenting symptoms and the patient is not reassured by the advice of several doctors. It is important to outrule any evidence of an underlying anxiety or depressive disorder on mental state examination and any possible malingering. Multiple physical symptoms in someone over 40 years suggest a primary diagnosis of depressive disorder; in this case the woman is younger. **[I. pp. 162–5]**

343 **Answer: D.** Latah is a culture-bound dissociative state in the Far East and North Africa mainly presenting with echolalia, automatic obedience and hysterical reaction to stress. It is more common in women. **[H. p. 387]**

344 **Answer: B.** Patient A displays thought broadcast and possibly thought insertion. Patient C has had a delusional perception, a delusional interpretation of a normal perception which has great meaning for the patient. Patient D is experiencing made emotion while patient E has arguing voices discussing him in the third person. Patient B demonstrates a bizarre delusion and neologisms which are both suggestive of schizophrenia but are not first-rank symptoms. **[D. pp. 151–4]**

345 Which one of the following is not compatible with the concept of pseudohallucinations?

A. They may occur in healthy individuals.

B. Patients have control over them.

C. Patients recognise that they are not 'real'.

D. They may coexist with hallucinations.

E. They do not occur spontaneously.

346 A 35-year-old married woman is referred for assessment by her GP who reports that she is having sexual difficulties. She is physically well. The patient reports that she and her husband both enjoy an intimate relationship but have been unable to achieve penetration. Which of the following is the most likely diagnosis?

A. Female orgasmic disorder.

B. Female sexual arousal disorder.

C. Hypoactive sexual desire disorder.

D. Sexual aversion disorder.

E. Vaginismus.

347 A 59-year-old male with a 30-year history of paranoid schizophrenia has developed tardive dyskinesia (TD). Which of the following treatments is most likely to improve this man's TD?

A. Change to an atypical antipsychotic.

B. Commence clozapine.

C. Discontinue antipsychotic medication.

D. Reduce the dose of the antipsychotic.

E. Stop anti-cholinergic medication.

348 A 28-year-old man of Asian origin has a 25 g weight attached by a string to the end of his penis. When questioned regarding this by his new and somewhat alarmed girlfriend he looks anxious and mumbles something about wanting 'to make it bigger'. He then says to forget what he has just said: he claims that it is a new range of jewellery that is all the rage in Germany. She suspects he is telling her lies. What may be the problem?

A. Amok.   B. Koro.

C. Latah.   D. Voodoo.

E. Windigo.

345 **Answer: E.** There is no agreed definition of pseudohallucination. Modern literature uses the term to describe a percept which arises spontaneously, is somewhat controllable and is recognised by the subject as being a product of their own mentation. The term also indicates that the percept is of altered (usually heightened) intensity compared to voluntarily imagined percepts. They may occur in healthy individuals. Interestingly, Kurt Schneider believed that *Gedankenlautwerden* were a transitional phenomenon between auditory hallucinations, difficult-to-control thoughts and a very vivid imagination. Using this definition *Gedankenlautwerden* may be a pseudohallucination. **[M. p. 57; T. p. 85]**

346 **Answer: E.** Sexual disorders can be categorised into those affecting sexual desire, affecting sexual arousal, affecting orgasm and causing pain. Vaginismus is a recurrent or persistent involuntary spasm of the musculature of the outer third of the vagina which interferes with sexual intercourse. It is the only one of the female sexual disorders which prevents completion of sexual intercourse. **[AG. pp. 488–90; AH. pp. 245–50]**

347 **Answer: B.** Clozapine is the most likely antipsychotic to be associated with resolution of tardive dyskinesia symptoms. **[AQ. p. 72]**

348 **Answer: B.** All are culture-bound syndromes. Koro involves the fear that the penis will shrink back into his abdomen (sometimes further into the chest or brain) and will kill the person. Weights on strings such as that described can be purchased in some countries where koro is found. Latah is described in Malaysia and involves suggestibility and automatic obedience. Voodoo has been described in Haiti and involves fear of death if a taboo is broken. Amok, also seen in Malaysia, is associated with depersonalisation and acts of rage. Windigo involves a fear of becoming a cannibal, found among some Canadian Indians. **[D. pp. 238–9]**

349 A patient is suffering from insomnia and other physical problems for which he is on a long list of medications (given below). Which one of them is least likely to cause insomnia?

A. Aminophylline.

B. Clonidine.

C. Dothiepin.

D. Paracetamol.

E. Reboxetine.

350 A patient with schizophrenia describes hearing a voice telling him to 'go home' when he hears the kettle start to boil at work. The voice is not his own and it is uncontrollable. Which of the following best describes his experience?

A. Auditory hallucination.

B. Autoscopic auditory hallucination.

C. Extracampine auditory hallucination.

D. Functional auditory hallucination.

E. Reflex auditory hallucination.

351 A 55-year-old patient being treated for depression has shown very little response to medication. Which of the following factors would be the strongest predictor of a positive response to ECT for this man?

A. Delusions.

B. Hypochondriacal symptoms.

C. Personality disorder.

D. Previous response to ECT.

E. Psychomotor retardation.

352 A 32-year-old woman is referred by her GP to you for investigation of unusual gait. She has also been referred to a neurologist and physical investigations are all normal. When asked to walk, she exhibits a gait that changes from festinant to a waddling gait and then to a drunken stagger. What is the most likely diagnosis in this case?

A. Cerebellar disorder.

B. Dissociative motor disorder.

C. Parkinson's disease.

D. Posterior column lesion.

E. Proximal myopathy.

349 **Answer: C.** Dothiepin has sedative effect, while all other options given in this question can cause insomnia. Other common medications that cause insomnia include: SSRIs, MAOIs, venlafaxine, anti-Parkinsonian medication, chemotherapy agents and thyroxine. **[AB. p. 393]**

350 **Answer: D.** Autoscopy is the experience of seeing oneself and knowing that it is oneself. Extracampine hallucinations are where the hallucinations are outside the normal limits of the sensory fields. Reflex hallucinations are where a stimulus in one sensory modality triggers a hallucination in another modality. Functional hallucinations are where the triggering stimulus and the hallucination occur in the same modality. **[T. p. 85]**

351 **Answer: D.** Hypochondriasis and personality disorder are two negative predictors of response to ECT. Psychomotor retardation and delusions are positive predictors. However, a history of previous response to ECT is the most robust predictor of all. **[S. pp. 602–3]**

352 **Answer: B.** In this case, as all investigations are normal, it cannot be any of the physical causes mentioned (i.e. cerebellar lesion – drunken gait, proximal myopathy – waddling gait, Parkinsonian – festinant gait). A posterior column lesion results in a gait where there is clumsy slapping down of the feet on a broad base. Hence the answer is a dissociative motor disorder. **[I. p. 159; AO. p. 370]**

353 All of the following are predisposing and/or associated factors for phobic disorders except:

A. Chaotic families.

B. Equal social class distribution.

C. History of childhood enuresis.

D. Major life events.

E. Sexual problems in female patients.

354 A patient has been diagnosed with panic disorder. From the list below, which is the least likely organic differential diagnosis for panic disorder?

A. Carcinoid syndrome.

B. Cushing's disease.

C. Hyperparathyroidism.

D. Hypoglycaemia.

E. Parkinson's disease.

355 A patient complains that she worries all the time that her children will come to some harm. She has distressing images of herself hitting them. The imagery is abhorrent to her and she used to resist the thoughts. Now she counts to 100 in her head. Although she recognises the thoughts and images are senseless she feels that she must do this to protect them from harm and to decrease her anxiety. The psychopathological term best describing this is?

A. Cotard's syndrome.

B. Delusional thinking.

C. Obsessional thoughts and images with covert compulsion.

D. Obsessional thoughts and images with overt compulsion.

E. Overvalued idea.

356 Which of the following is not an indication for electroconvulsive therapy?

A. Mania.

B. Neuroleptic malignant syndrome.

C. Obsessive compulsive disorder.

D. Parkinson's disease.

E. Schizophrenia.

353 Answer: A. Predisposing and/or associated factors for phobic disorders include the following: passive, anxious and dependent personality traits, stable families, history of childhood fears and enuresis and higher incidents of sexual problems in females. There is no difference from the general population in regard to education and social class. **[H. pp. 67–8]**

354 Answer: E. Parkinson's disease is not a differential diagnosis for panic disorder, while all other illnesses listed can mimic panic disorder, the most common being hyperthyroidism and phaeochromocytoma **[AB. p. 345]**

355 Answer: C. Obsessions are intrusive thoughts, images or impulses which are involuntary and automatic and give rise to anxiety. They are recognised as being products of the patient's own mind and are usually resisted. Compulsions are voluntary activities either physical or mental (covert) which decrease the anxiety temporarily and therefore act to maintain the cycle. In this case the patient has an obsessional thought that her children will come to some harm. The compulsion is counting in her head. It is not a delusion because she knows it is not real. It is not an overvalued idea because she realises it is senseless. **[T. p. 88; Salkovskis P, Forrester E, Richards C. Cognitive-behavioural approach to understanding obsessional thinking, *British Journal of Psychiatry*. 1998; 173: 53–63]**

356 Answer: C. An acute response to ECT has been demonstrated in OCD, but patients soon relapsed and ECT is not recommended for this disorder. The use of ECT in mania is reserved for patients who are resistant or intolerant to the usual medication treatments or who have severe symptoms, for example manic delirium. Neuroleptic malignant syndrome shows outcomes with ECT which are equivalent to those obtained pharmacologically. Schizophrenia is the second commonest indication for ECT, although there is a lack of consensus about its use in this disorder. Motor symptoms in Parkinson's disease have been shown to be lessened by ECT, with effects lasting four to six weeks. **[P. pp. 2972–4]**

357 Which of the following is not a neurotransmitter produced by the human body?

A. Anandamide.

B. Beta endorphin.

C. Cannabinoid.

D. Neuropeptide Y.

E. Substance P.

358 Regarding service users who present with deliberate self-harm, all of the following are correct except:

A. 1% of them will commit suicide in the first year after presentation.

B. 10% of them ultimately commit suicide.

C. 50% of repeated deliberate self-harm is by drug overdose.

D. 50% of suicides in general have history of deliberate self-harm.

E. Recent alcohol intake is associated for many self-harmers.

359 Regarding the epidemiology of anxiety disorders, which of the following disorders is less likely to be over-represented among females?

A. Agoraphobia.

B. Generalised anxiety disorder.

C. Panic disorder.

D. Simple phobia.

E. Social phobia.

360 Which of the following terms best describes where a patient with schizophrenia moves his limbs or body in response to light pressure from the examiner?

A. Advertence.

B. *Mitmachen.*

C. Negativism.

D. *Schnauzkrampf.*

E. Waxy flexibility.

357 **Answer: C.** Anandamide is a lipid neurotransmitter and is described as the brain's own marijuana. Cannabinoids are not produced by the human brain. Beta endorphin is the brain's own opiate. **[AR. p. 18]**

358 **Answer: C.** Approximately 90% of repeated deliberate self-harm is by drug overdose, not 50%. Recent alcohol intake has been found in 50% of males and between 25 and 45% in females. Predictors of repetition include: previous suicidal behaviour, personality disorder, history of violence and alcohol dependence. **[H. pp. 155–6]**

359 **Answer: E.** Social phobia is equally common among males and females, while all other anxiety disorders are noticed to be more common in women as compared to men. **[AB. pp. 344–56]**

360 **Answer: B.** Advertence is an abnormal movement in schizophrenia whereby a patient turns to face someone addressing him in an exaggerated, inflexible and bizarre manner. Negativism is where a patient actively resists all attempts to make contact with him. *Schnauzkrampf* is a facial grimace whereby the lips and nose are brought together in a pout. Waxy flexibility is where the patient's body can be manipulated into a posture which the patient then maintains for a sustained period. **[D. p. 337]**

361 Which of the following features is not characteristic of a hypnotic state?

A. Acceptance of distortions.

B. Attention is indiscriminately directed.

C. Diminished reality testing.

D. Increased suggestibility.

E. Post-hypnotic amnesia.

362 A 33-year-old married housewife and mother of a one-year-old child has a diagnosis of obsessive compulsive disorder. Which of the following activities of daily living are most likely to cause her difficulty in rearing her child?

A. Counting.

B. Fears of contamination.

C. Insistence on symmetry.

D. Obsessional doubting.

E. Washing.

363 Which of the following is less likely to be associated with increased risk of suicide?

A. Alcoholism.

B. Incarceration in prison.

C. Physical illness.

D. Religious affiliation.

E. Unemployment.

364 Jane's mother died in a car crash a few weeks ago. Which of the following is the best predicator of development of depressive disorder following bereavement?

A. History of cannabis use.

B. Large homogeneous family.

C. Previous death in family.

D. Social class VI.

E. Traumatic death.

361 **Answer: B.** The characteristics of a hypnotic state have been described as follows:

- The subject ceases to make his or her own plans.
- Attention is selectively directed, for example towards the voice of the hypnotist.
- Reality testing is decreased and distortions are accepted.
- Suggestibility is increased.
- The subject readily enacts unusual roles.
- Post-hypnotic amnesia is often present.

[D. p. 47]

362 **Answer: E.** Rasmussen and Tsaung found checking compulsions to be the commonest symptoms (63%) in OCD, followed by washing (50%) and fears of contamination (45%). **[N. pp. 69–70]**

363 **Answer: D.** Religious affiliation is a protective factor against suicide. On the other hand alcoholism, psychiatric morbidity, personality disorder, physical illness and being a prison inmate are all associated with increased rates of suicide. **[H. pp. 150–2]**

364 **Answer: E.** A traumatic death is a risk factor for development of depression following bereavement. Other predictors are: previous history of depression, intense grief or depressive symptoms early in the grief reaction, poor social support and little experience of death. All the other options given in the question are distracters. **[AB. p. 366]**

365 Which one of the following statements concerning schizophrenia is false?

    A. Ideas of reference occur in 90% of cases.

    B. Lifetime suicide risk is 10%.

    C. The sex ratio is equal.

    D. Thought alienation occurs in 52% of cases.

    E. Urban populations have a higher prevalence than rural populations.

366 A 35-year-old man with schizophrenia reports that he has realised that he is being targeted by a terrorist organisation which is accessing his thoughts through the Internet. When asked what makes him think this he replies that he does not 'think' it, but that it is true. He says that the realisation came to him 'out of the blue'. Which of the following options best describes this man's experience?

    A. Autochthonous delusion.

    B. Delusional memory.

    C. Delusional mood.

    D. Delusional percept.

    E. Nihilistic delusions.

367 Which of the following psychosurgeries is no longer carried out to treat psychiatric illness?

    A. Capsulotomy.

    B. Cingulotomy.

    C. Limbic leucotomy.

    D. Subcaudate tractomy.

    E. Trepanation.

368 Which of the following is most correct with respect to logoclonia?

    A. It is a disorder of speech in schizophrenia.

    B. It is synonymous with echolalia.

    C. It is synonymous with palilalia.

    D. It is synonymous with verbigeration.

    E. It is the spastic repetition of syllables.

365 **Answer: A.** According to the IPSS survey from the WHO, ideas of reference occur in 70% of cases. **[T. p. 246]**

366 **Answer: A.** The patient is describing an autochthonous delusion or delusional intuition, which occurs out of the blue to the patient. Delusional intuition occurs in one stage, unlike a delusional percept which occurs in two stages: perception followed by false interpretation. Delusional mood refers to a feeling of anticipation that something significant is going to happen. The patient feels perplexed, apprehensive and uncomfortable. It is followed by the formation of a delusion, and tends to occur in the early development of a schizophrenic illness. Delusional memory occurs when the patient recounts as remembered an event or idea that is delusional in nature. It has the characteristics of a delusional percept or delusional intuition but is remembered from the past rather than in the present. These terms all refer to the form of the delusion. Nihilistic refers to the content of the delusion and describes an extreme negative attitude. **[D. pp. 104–11, 121]**

367 **Answer: E.** Trepanation is no longer carried as a psychosurgery to relieve the symptoms of mental illness. From Neolithic times to the Middle Ages, trepanation was performed. The other psychosurgeries listed are still being used as last-resort treatments for intractable depressive, anxiety, and obsessive compulsive disorders. **[G. pp. 216–17]**

368 **Answer: E.** Logoclonia is the spastic repetition of syllables: the last syllable of the last word is repeated. In palilalia the whole word is repeated. They occur in organic brain disorders such as Parkinsonism and Alzheimer's disease. Speech disorders in schizophrenia include mutism, echolalia and verbigeration. Verbigeration is a stereotyped repeating of the same words or phrases: it may continue for prolonged periods. **[M. p. 63, D. p. 158, E. p. 1184]**

369 A man who has been serving in the army for years has recently returned from the war in Iraq. His GP thinks he is suffering from post-traumatic stress disorder. Which of his symptoms below is not a symptom of post-traumatic stress disorder according to ICD-10?

A. Amnesia for the trauma.

B. Avoidance.

C. Hypervigilance.

D. Reliving the trauma.

E. Suicidal thoughts.

370 Regarding the dopamine hypothesis of schizophrenia, which one of the following statements is false?

A. Amphetamine causes synaptical release of dopamine and causes psychotic symptoms.

B. Disulfiram inhibits dopamine metabolism and exacerbates schizophrenia.

C. Lysergic acid diethylamide is a D_4 agonist and causes hallucinations.

D. Only the flupenthixol isomer that is a D_2 antagonist is an effective antipsychotic.

E. PET scans reveal asymmetrical D_2 receptor concentrations in schizophrenic patients.

371 A patient with schizophrenia shows marked disturbance of speech. While the words he uses are recognisable they are so disorganised in sentences that they are meaningless. Which of the following speech disorders is this man demonstrating?

A. Cluttering.

B. Echolalia.

C. Logoclonia.

D. Palilalia.

E. Paragrammatism.

372 Which of the following is not one of the four humours described as part of the humour theory to explain both physical and mental illnesses?

A. Blood.

B. Black bile.

C. Phlegm.

D. Urine.

E. Yellow bile.

369 **Answer: E.** Suicidal thoughts are not listed as a symptom of post-trauma stress disorder, but of course can happen in depressive disorder, which is a comorbid condition. Other symptoms of post-traumatic stress disorder according to ICD 10 are: difficulty falling or staying asleep, irritability, difficulty in concentration and hypervigilance. **[AB. p. 368]**

370 **Answer: C.** LSD is a $5HT_{2a/2c}$ receptor agonist. **[T. p. 255]**

371 **Answer: E.** Paragrammatism refers to the disorder of grammatical construction. In schizophrenia it is termed word salad. Cluttering is a disturbance of fluency involving an abnormally rapid rate and erratic rhythm of speech that impedes intelligibility. In echolalia the patient repeats words or parts of sentences that are spoken to him or in his presence. It most often occurs in excited schizophrenic states, with learning disability and with organic states. Logoclonia describes the spastic repetition of syllables that occurs in Parkinsonism. Palilalia is the repetition of a word or phrase. It is a perseveration phenomenon. **[P. pp. 849–59; D. pp. 158–9]**

372 **Answer: D.** Urine is not one of the four humours. The humour theory is a theory of physiology in which the state of health and by extension the state of mind, or character, depended upon a balance among the four elemental fluids: blood, yellow bile, phlegm, and black bile. **[AT. pp. 5–7]**

373 Which is the least correct statement regarding homosexuality?

A. 1% of men are only attracted to other men.

B. Boarding-school education increases the possibility one will be homosexual in later life.

C. First sexual experience tends to be at a later age among homosexual people.

D. If you are of a higher socioeconomic group it is more likely you have had homosexual activity at some time.

E. Men in Greater London are twice as likely to have had homosexual sexual activity as men anywhere else in Great Britain.

374 A person has been referred to your outpatient clinic with the diagnosis of dissocial personality disorder. You check ICD-10 for the diagnostic criteria. From the list below, which is the most likely finding?

A. Emotionally cold.

B. History of childhood conduct disorder.

C. Interpersonal discomfort.

D. Self-conscious.

E. Unpredictable affect.

375 Which one of the following is false regarding the diagnosis of ICD-10 schizophrenia?

A. Positive symptoms such as hallucinations must be present for at least one month.

B. Running commentary occurring alone is sufficient for the diagnosis.

C. Symptoms of simple schizophrenia for six months are sufficient for its diagnosis.

D. Thought insertion occurring alone is sufficient for the diagnosis.

E. Thought disorder alone is not sufficient to diagnose paranoid schizophrenia.

376 Which of the following medications acts primarily by modifying serotonin degradation?

A. Clomipramine.

B. Fluoxetine.

C. Mirtazapine.

D. Phenelzine.

E. Venlafaxine.

373 **Answer: B.** Boarding-school education increases your likelihood to experience homosexual activity but has little effect on later life. All the other statements are true. **[R. p. 443]**

374 **Answer: B.** Other common symptoms present are:

- callous lack of concern for others
- irresponsibility
- irritability
- aggression
- inability to maintain enduring relationships
- disregard and violation of others' rights.

Schizoid personality is associated with emotionally cold response. **[AB. p. 447]**

375 **Answer: C.** Simple schizophrenia requires the presence of symptoms for at least one year. **[I. pp. 86–90]**

376 **Answer: D.** Phenelzine is a monoamine oxidase inhibitor. Monamine oxidase oxidises most serotonin to 5-hydroxyindoleacetaldehyde. It is then broken down to 5-hydroxyindoleacetic acid (5-HIAA) by aldehyde dehydrogenase: this is the major metabolite of serotonin degradation. Fluoxetine acts as a selective serotonin reuptake inhibitor. Clomipramine inhibits the reuptake of serotonin and its metabolite desmethylclomipramine inhibits the reuptake of noradrenaline. Mirtazapine is a noradrenergic and specific serotonergic antidepressant, which acts by inhibiting α_2 receptors to specifically increase serotonin at the $5HT_{1A}$ receptor and increase noradrenergic transmission. Venlafaxine is a serotonin and noradrenaline reuptake inhibitor at medium to high doses **[A. pp. 62–74, 420]**

377 A 55-year-old woman attends your new patient clinic complaining of depressive symptoms. You diagnose a moderate depressive episode. This woman's preference is for psychotherapy. You suggest cognitive behaviour therapy. Which of the following is not part of CBT?

A. Challenging 'logical errors'.

B. Focus on the 'here and now'.

C. Focus on the relationship with the therapist.

D. Homework tasks.

E. Use of problem solving.

378 Regarding schizophrenia, which of the following theories is still useful?

A. Abnormal family communication.

B. Double bind.

C. Expressed emotion.

D. Marital skew and marital schism.

E. Schizophrenogenic mother.

379 A 55-year-old woman has been diagnosed with psychotic illness for the first time. Her diagnosis is paraphrenia. From the list below, which feature is the most prominent in this presentation?

A. Bizarre behaviour.

B. Blunted affect.

C. Change in personality.

D. Formal thought disorder.

E. Hallucinations.

380 According to Andreasen, which one of the following is not a positive symptom of schizophrenia?

A. Aggressive behaviour.

B. Derailment.

C. Inappropriate affect.

D. Stereotyped behaviour.

E. Thought blocking.

377 **Answer: C.** The relationship with the therapist is of lesser importance in CBT. [**www.trickcyclists.co.uk/OSCEs/**]

378 **Answer: C.** Historically, the following types of family dysfunctions were at various times believed to be a cause of schizophrenia: schizophrenogenic mother, double bind, marital skew and marital schism and abnormal family communication. These theories are now out of favour, but there is evidence for the more recent theory relating to the effect of expressed emotion with respect to relapse in schizophrenia. [**R. pp. 137–8**]

379 **Answer: E.** Paraphrenia was first described by Kraepelin. It is characterised by delusions and hallucinations while other symptoms like blunted affect, formal thought disorder or change in personality are not prominent. [**AB. p. 480**]

380 **Answer: E.** This is a component of alogia, a negative symptom. The other groups of negative symptoms are: affective flattening/blunting, avolition-apathy, anhedonia-asociality, and attentional difficulties. [**T. p. 247**]

381 A 55-year-old patient with a history of depression tells you that she is planning to go out for a meal to celebrate her birthday. She is currently taking phenelzine. Which of the following foods is safest for this woman to order?

A. Brie cheese.

B. Caviar.

C. Guacamole.

D. Pheasant.

E. Sausages.

382 A 40-year-old female patient with schizophrenia, recently admitted to the acute psychiatric unit where you work, describes to you looking in the mirror and not seeing her own image. She is very frightened by this. What term best describes this phenomenon?

A. Autoscopy.

B. Eidetic image.

C. Negative autoscopy.

D. Sosia illusion.

E. Subjective doubles.

383 Lithium is less likely to be effective in which of the following conditions?

A. Augmentation in resistant depression.

B. Maintenance therapy for bipolar disorder.

C. Prophylaxis for bipolar disorder.

D. Prophylaxis for unipolar disorder.

E. Treatment of mania.

384 David has attended sessions with the alcohol counsellor for the last year. He always thought that his depression was responsible for his drinking. Today for the first time he accepted that he has a problem with drinking and can appreciate both negative and positive aspects of alcohol. In terms of stages of change, at what stage is David at present?

A. Action.

B. Contemplation.

C. Decision.

D. Maintenance.

E. Pre-contemplation.

381 **Answer: E.** When taking MAOIs it is important to avoid tyramine-containing foods because of the risk of hypertensive crisis. The patient must also avoid foods that are matured or may be spoiling. Soft mature cheeses, guacamole and caviar all contain levels of tyramine which should be avoided. Pheasant is a game fowl which is hung and may be spoiled. Sausages have been found to contain only minute amounts of tyramine and are not considered a particular risk. [**X. pp. 300–1**]

382 **Answer: C.** Autoscopy is a visual hallucination of oneself, i.e. the doppelganger phenomenon. Negative autoscopy is when on reflection of oneself in a mirror no image is seen. Sosia illusion is where one's spouse, along with other people, are doubles. Subjective doubles is where an individual believes that another individual has been transformed into his own self. An eidetic image is a recollection of a memory with a vivid perception. [**F. pp. 85–7**]

383 **Answer: D.** Lithium is used as a treatment of mania, prophylaxis for bipolar disorder, maintenance therapy in bipolar disorder and in augmentation in cases of resistant depression. It may also be useful in schizoaffective disorder and for treating aggressive/impulsive behaviour. It is not recommended as a first-line drug in prophylaxis for unipolar disorder. [**N. p. 279**]

384 **Answer: B.** There are various stages of change and harm reduction starting from pre-contemplation, which is basically denial of the problem, followed by contemplation where the person accepts that he has a problem with a particular drug. At decision stage, the user decides on whether to continue or attempt change. This stage is followed by action, when the user attempts change. At maintenance, the user tries to improve areas of life harmed by drug use. The last stage is relapse with return of previous behaviours. [**AB. p. 503**]

385 Crow described an increase in the number of dopamine receptors in the brains of many deceased patients with schizophrenic illnesses. Along with other characteristics he named this group 'Type 1'. Which one of the following is not a characteristic of this group?

A. Acute schizophrenia.

B. No intellectual impairment.

C. Poor response to neuroleptics.

D. Reversible.

E. Symptoms of delusions and hallucinations.

386 A 22-year-old woman working as an administrative manager is referred by her GP who reports that she is suicidal. She is accompanied by her parents with whom she has a good relationship. The patient tells you that she has been feeling depressed for about three months and has been feeling worse in the last two weeks. She has never harmed herself in the past. Which of this patient's characteristics would increase your concern regarding her suicidal risk?

A. Employment status.   B. Gender.

C. Socioeconomic group.   D. Mental illness.

E. Social support.

387 Stopping when a red light is displayed at a traffic light is an example of what type of learning?

A. Avoidance learning.   B. Chaining.

C. Latent learning.   D. One-trial learning.

E. Shaping.

388 Which of the following is least associated with contributing to the understanding of schizophrenia?

A. Cameron.   B. Cade.

C. Bleuler.   D. Goldstein.

E. Kraepelin.

385 **Answer: C.** Crow's Type 1 schizophrenia tends to respond well to neuroleptics. The postulated pathological process in Type 2 schizophrenia is cell loss with structural changes. **[T. p. 247]**

386 **Answer: D.** The factors for increased risk of suicide include male gender, lack of social support, unemployment, lower socioeconomic category (especially for those in a middle age group), severe mental illness (especially depression) and a history of self-harm. This woman's mental illness is her most significant risk factor. **[R. p. 400]**

387 **Answer: A.** This is a situation where no aversive stimulus is presented if a suitable action is taken. Chaining and shaping are parts of operant conditioning. Shaping involves successive approximations to the desired behaviour. Chaining is where a complex behaviour is broken down into a series of simpler steps, taught separately and then linked together. Latent learning is learning occurring in the absence of changes in behaviour. One-trial learning is a conditioned reflex based on the single pairing of the conditioned stimulus and unconditioned stimulus. **[C. pp. 124, 129–30; F. pp. 3–4]**

388 **Answer: B.** Bleuler coined the term 'schizophrenia' and also described it as being associated with the following: loosening of associations, affective flattening, autism and ambivalence. Cameron postulated the term 'over-inclusive thinking' while Goldstein viewed schizophrenia's thought disorder as concrete thinking. Kraepelin is associated with the term 'dementia praecox'. John Cade's contribution was the introduction of lithium as a treatment for mania in 1949. **[H. pp. 19, 328]**

389 Diana drinks four pints of beer (4% alcohol by volume) twice weekly. She also takes three measures of vodka (37.5% alcohol by volume) on Saturday. How many alcohol units is she consuming in a week?

A. 7

B. 11.

C. 15

D. 19.

E. 21.

390 Liddle studied regional cerebral activity of patients with chronic schizophrenia using PET scans and neuropsychological testing. On factor analysis he discovered three distinct sub-syndromes with their own characteristic blood flow. Which one of the following statements is true?

A. Distractibility is a component of the *reality distortion syndrome*.

B. Poverty of speech is a component of the *disorganisation syndrome*.

C. The *disorganisation syndrome* is associated with increased activity in the right cingulate and dorsomedial thalamic nuclei.

D. The *psychomotor poverty syndrome* is associated with increased blood flow in the prefrontal lobe.

E. The *reality distortion syndrome* is associated with decreased flow in the temporal lobe (especially the hippocampal regions).

391 A 44-year-old man is seen with depression. He is commenced on escitalopram 10 mg daily. After six weeks he has shown no response to treatment. What is the next step in this man's biological management?

A. Add bupropion.

B. Add lithium.

C. Change to an alternative antidepressant.

D. Consider ECT.

E. Increase the dose of escitalopram.

392 A 29-year-old female patient in A&E has the following signs and symptoms: nausea, vomiting, increased blood pressure and papilloedema. There is no history of trauma or pyrexia in this case. The casualty officer asks you, the duty psychiatrist, for an opinion of the most likely diagnosis in this case. Would it be?

A. Head injury.

B. Meningeal infection.

C. Non-communicating hydrocephalus.

D. Marchiafava-Bignami disease.

E. Subacute combined degeneration of the cord.

389 **Answer: D.** The formula to calculate the number of units is volume in litres multiplied by percentage of alcohol. Usually each pint of beer contains two units of alcohol while a single measure of spirits is one unit of alcohol. So, Diana is drinking 19 units per week. **[AB. p. 513]**

390 **Answer: C.** Distractibility is in fact a component of the disorganisation syndrome, whereas poverty of speech is a component of the psychomotor poverty syndrome. The psychomotor poverty syndrome is associated with decreased blood flow to the prefrontal regions and the reality distortion syndrome is associated with increased blood flow to the left temporal lobe. **[R. p. 371]**

391 **Answer: E.** If the patient fails to respond to the average dose of an antidepressant, provided he is tolerating the medication, he should first be prescribed a higher dose. If there is still no improvement in a further two weeks, an alternative antidepressant should be considered. If following an adequate trial of the alternative antidepressant at an adequate dose he still shows no improvement, treatments for refractory depression should be considered. **[V. p. 187]**

392 **Answer: C.** Symptoms that occur with a non-communicating hydrocephalus are nausea, vomiting, increased blood pressure and papilloedema. Non-communicating hydrocephalus and increased intracranial pressure are caused by flow obstruction in the third or fourth ventricle. A reduced pulse and headache worse on lying down are also signs. Head injury and meningeal infection can be outruled as there is no evidence of trauma or pyrexia in this scenario. Meningeal infection would give a similar clinical picture. Marchiafava-Bignami disease is a complication of alcohol dependence: it involves degeneration of the corpus callosum with clinical symptoms of recurrent seizures and dementia. Subacute combined degeneration of the cord is due to vitamin B_{12} deficiency and presents with ataxic gait, upper motor neuron signs in the lower limbs, along with dementia and peripheral neuropathy. **[AF. p. 27; H. p. 126; AO. pp. 376–7]**

393 Which of the following is not a parietal lobe function?

A. Ability to draw a clock face

B. Ability to localise body parts.

C. Ability to name fingers.

D. Comprehension of words.

E. Right-left orientation.

394 Alan has been diagnosed with alcohol dependence syndrome. His father also had the same problem. From the list below, which statement is true regarding genetics and alcoholism?

A. Adopted children of alcoholic patients have the same risk as the general population.

B. First-degree relatives of alcoholics have ten times higher risk than the general population.

C. Oriental people drink less than European people.

D. The gene for alcoholism has been identified on chromosome 22.

E. The risk of developing alcoholism is the same in identical and non-identical twins.

395 Which one of the following statements regarding the size of the cerebral ventricles of patients with schizophrenia is true?

A. They are equal in size in discordant monozygotic twins.

B. They are increased in size at disease onset.

C. They are reduced in size at disease onset.

D. They decrease in size as the disorder progresses.

E. They increase in size as the disorder progresses.

396 A 45-year-old woman attending your service has been diagnosed with depression. However, she has shown little response to her antidepressant medication. She has been on escitalopram 5 mg for six weeks with no response. She complains of loss of libido since commencing on the medication. She is also taking cimetidine. What is the likely cause of treatment resistance in this woman's case?

A. Drug interactions.

B. Inadequate dosage of antidepressant.

C. Insufficient time for antidepressant to be effective.

D. Non-compliance.

E. Unaddressed psychiatric comorbidity.

393 **Answer: D.** The parietal lobe can be checked by testing the ability to copy an asymmetrical object, to draw a clock face, to construct a star from matchsticks and to test right-left orientation. Parietal lobe functions include the ability to name fingers; however, the comprehension of words is part of temporal lobe function. **[N. p. 152]**

394 **Answer: C.** The metabolically inactive form of alcohol dehydrogenase is common in oriental people. It leads to accumulation of acetaldehyde and the unpleasant flushing which results in lower rates of alcohol problems in those populations. First-degree relatives have double the risk of alcohol problems and identical twins have significantly higher rates compared to non-identical twins. There is no identified single gene for alcoholism and it is expected to have polygenic inheritance. **[AB. p. 507]**

395 **Answer: B.** Cerebral ventricles are enlarged at disease onset but this does not progress. It is only apparent in the affected monozygotic twin. **[T. p. 254]**

396 **Answer: B.** This woman has been taking only 5 mg of escitalopram, albeit for an adequate period of six weeks. The recommended dose for the treatment of depression is 10 mg daily, increasing to a maximum of 20 mg. Loss of libido is a potential side-effect of escitalopram, indicating that this patient is compliant with her medication. Escitalopram has a low likelihood of drug interaction and so the co-prescription of cimetidine is unlikely to be causing a difficulty. **[X. pp. 54, 279]**

397 A 37-year-old Chinese man is assessed by you complaining of abdominal pain, low energy and poor interest. Using ICD-10 criteria you diagnose a current depressive episode. You are certain of your diagnosis. Which of the following terms describes the difficulty that arises when a Western psychiatric diagnostic category is improperly used in a culture in which the category has no relevance?

A. Cultural fallacy.

B. Ecological fallacy.

C. Koro.

D. Transcultural psychiatry.

E. Transcultural uncertainty.

398 Which of the following is a component of insight?

A. All of the items below.

B. Attribution of illness.

C. Awareness of social consequences of illness.

D. Awareness of treatment.

E. Recognition of illness.

399 A patient has alcohol dependence syndrome and has started disulfiram. From the list below, what might most be a contraindication of disulfiram?

A. Asian race.

B. Severe depression.

C. Poor family support.

D. Priapism.

E. Psychotic symptoms.

400 Which one of the following statements regarding structural brain abnormalities in schizophrenia is false?

A. Gliosis is frequently found.

B. The cortical volume is decreased.

C. The parahippocampus is smaller.

D. The thalamus is smaller.

E. The ventricles are larger.

397 **Answer: A.** The term *cultural fallacy* is used to describe the difficulty that arises when a Western psychiatric diagnostic category is improperly used in a culture in which the category has no relevance. Ecological fallacy is a statistical term used to describe the fallacy that assumes that phenomena described at a macro (i.e. national) level will hold true at a micro (i.e. individual) level. Koro is a specific culture-bound syndrome. D and E are distracters. **[E. p. 464; A. p. 189]**

398 **Answer: A.** Most authors would consider insight to not be a binary concept, i.e. it is not just either 'present' or 'absent'. Various components of insight are described such as those listed in items B to E. **[N. pp. 21–2]**

399 **Answer: E.** Disulfiram is an irreversible inhibitor of acetaldehyde dehydrogenase and there are reports of psychotic reactions with disulfiram, therefore it is better avoided in patients with a history of psychotic symptoms. All other options given here are distracters. **[AB. p. 522]**

400 **Answer: A.** Consistent findings are reduced brain volume, disproportionately reduced temporal lobes (including the hippocampi), reduced thalami and increased ventricular volume. Gliosis was reported by Alzheimer but has not subsequently been confirmed. **[M. p. 608; T. p. 254]**

401 A 55-year-old man has a long history of schizophrenia. He is documented as having chronic schizophrenia with disorganisation syndrome, characterised by inappropriate affect, poverty of content of speech, tangentiality, derailment and distractibility. Who out of the following described this syndrome in chronic schizophrenia?

A. Andreasen.

B. Bleuler.

C. Crow.

D. Liddle.

E. Schneider.

402 You are a psychiatric SHO in your third year of training and are asked by your clinical supervisor to embark on a piece of serviced-based research in the department. You decide to enlist help in administering a diagnostic interview to a sample of outpatient attendees. Which of the following diagnostic interviews would you choose that can be administered by a non-clinician?

A. Catego Programme.

B. Diagnostic Interview Schedule.

C. Present State Examination.

D. Research Diagnostic Criteria.

E. Structured Clinical Interview for DSM-IV.

403 You are seeing a 40-year-old man with schizophrenia – catatonic type. He displays abnormal movements. Which of the following is least likely to occur in this patient?

A. Automatic obedience.

B. Chorea.

C. Echopraxia.

D. *Mitgehen*.

E. Negativism.

404 A patient has paranoid schizophrenia and is currently on antipsychotic medication. You are worried that he may have developed neuroleptic malignant syndrome. From the list below, what is the most likely scenario that would increase the risk of neuroleptic malignant syndrome?

A. Addition of anticholinergic agents.

B. Changing olanzapine to quetiapine.

C. Male patient as compared to female.

D. Relaxed patient as compared to agitated.

E. Slow increase in antipsychotic medication.

401 **Answer: D.** Liddle described three syndromes of chronic schizophrenia: psychomotor poverty syndrome, disorganisation syndrome and reality distortion syndrome. Andreasen divided schizophrenia into two syndromes, positive and negative, according to a set of validated diagnostic criteria. Crow described type 1 and type 2 syndromes on the basis of post mortem findings. Subsequently, research evidence showed that cognitive impairment and tardive dyskinesia occur most commonly in patients with type 2 syndrome and are infrequent in those with type 1 schizophrenia. Bleuler is known for describing the primary or fundamental symptoms of schizophrenia as the 'four As': autism, ambivalence, abnormal association, and affective abnormality. Schneider described the first-rank symptoms of schizophrenia, which he believed differentiated schizophrenia from similar illnesses. [S. pp. 259–60, 266–7]

402 **Answer: B.** The Diagnostic Interview Schedule was developed for large epidemiological surveys, is highly structured and can be administered by non-clinicians. The Composite International Diagnostic Interview is a combination of the Diagnostic Interview Schedule and the Present State Examination. Interviewers without a clinical background can also use it. The other four interviews schedules are for use by trained clinicians. [A. p. 158]

403 **Answer: B.** Chorea is a type of movement disorder in which the movement looks as if it were part of an intentional movement but is brief and jerky. The movements are not rhythmical. It is not associated with catatonic schizophrenia. [N. pp. 14–15]

404 **Answer: A.** Addition of lithium or anticholinergic agents can increase the risk of neuroleptic malignant syndrome. Female patients are at more risk as compared to male patients. Similarly, high-potency drugs carry more risk as compared to low-potency drugs such as quetiapine. Agitation and rapid initiation of antipsychotics are both risk factors for development of neuroleptic malignant syndrome. [AB. p. 868]

405 A 25-year-old man with a family history of schizophrenia is diagnosed with schizophrenia. Which one of the following statements is false?

A. Children adopted away from their schizophrenic mothers shortly after birth are at an increased risk of later developing the disorder themselves.

B. Children of normal individuals who are placed with adoptive parents who then develop schizophrenia are at an increased risk of developing schizophrenia themselves.

C. The most powerful risk factor for schizophrenia is a family history of the disorder.

D. Twin studies show a 1.7% probandwise concordance rate for ICD-10 schizophrenia in dizygotic twins.

E. Twin studies show a 42% probandwise concordance rate for ICD-10 schizophrenia in monozygotic twins.

406 A 35-year-old woman is referred for assessment by her GP who reports that she has been complaining of widespread pain for the last five months. She has complained of pain in various areas on both the right and left sides and above and below the waist. She additionally complains of fatigue, low mood and sleep disturbance. On examination she complains of tenderness in many areas, including the occiput, trapezius, gluteus, and knees. Physical investigations are normal. What is the most likely diagnosis in this woman's case?

A. Body dysmorphic disorder.   B. Fibromyalgia.

C. Hypochondriasis.   D. Rheumatoid arthritis.

E. Somatisation disorder.

407 A 55-year-old man with a diagnosis of alcohol dependence syndrome attends your clinic. He blames his wife for his alcohol dependence, not seeing that he has any responsibility in this. 'If only she would stop nagging me Doc, I wouldn't have to go the pub every night to get away from her. She gets off on nagging!' What is this tendency to blame our own behaviour on external rather than internal causes called?

A. Denial.   B. Displacement.

C. Distortion.   D. Fundamental attribution error.

E. Repression.

408 All of the following are compatible with autochthonous delusions except:

A. Delusional atmosphere.   B. Delusional mood.

C. Schizophrenia.   D. Sudden intuitions.

E. Underlying personal stress.

405 **Answer: B.** It was found that the children of normal individuals who are placed with adoptive parents who then develop schizophrenia are at no increased risk of developing schizophrenia themselves. This further supports the theory that it is genes rather than intra-family environment that causes familial aggregation of schizophrenia. However, the lack of complete concordance between monozygotic twins supports the sizeable importance of environment. **[M. p. 599]**

406 **Answer: B.** The primary symptom of fibromyalgia is widespread pain with tenderness at multiple specified anatomical sites for at least three months. The most common associated symptoms are fatigue, depression, sleep disturbances, and cognitive problems. Depression and anxiety often develop and exacerbate the condition. Body dysmorphic disorder involves preoccupation with an imagined defect in appearance. Hypochondriasis is characterised by preoccupation with fears of having, or the idea that one has, a serious disease based on the misinterpretation of bodily symptoms. The duration of disturbance is at least six months. In somatisation disorder the patient experiences persistent recurrent multiple physical symptoms starting in early adult life or earlier. There is usually a long history of inconclusive investigations and procedures and high rates of social and occupational impairment. The DSM-IV criteria require four pain symptoms, two gastro-intestinal symptoms, one sexual symptom, and one pseudoneurological symptom for the diagnosis. The diagnosis of rheumatoid arthritis will be assisted by the presence of morning stiffness, symmetrical arthritis at multiple joints and the presence of rheumatoid nodules. Positive rheumatoid factor is present in about 80% and there may also be changes on X-ray. **[K. p. 2178; AH. pp. 229–36]**

407 **Answer: D.** The fundamental attribution error states that individuals attribute their own behaviour to external causes but others' behaviour to internal causes. Denial, displacement, distortion and repression are Freudian defence mechanisms. **[F. p. 20; G. pp. 103–4]**

408 **Answer: E.** Autochthonous delusions are primary delusions that arise suddenly (not out of a stressful situation). They can be associated with a period of delusional mood preceding their formation. Underlying personal stress can lead to secondary delusions. **[N. p. 16]**

409 A young child gets excited whenever he sees his father's car. He is presented with other cars but he does not get excited. Of what is this an example?

A. Discrimination.

B. Extinction.

C. Law of effect.

D. Positive reinforcement.

E. Stimulus generalisation.

410 Based on the WHO 10-country study, which one of the following has not been implicated as a statistically significant prognostic variable for remission from episodes of schizophrenia?

A. Acute versus gradual onset.

B. Age.

C. Developed/developing countries.

D. Duration of Untreated Psychosis (DUP).

E. Gender.

411 A 45-year-old Indian man is referred by his general practitioner for assessment. He recently arrived in the country and is very anxious, worrying about various aches and pains in his body. On further interview the patient states that his urine has turned whiter in colour. He feels tired most of the time and reveals that he feels very guilty. When questioned regarding the cause of his guilt he eventually states that he has been masturbating excessively. Which of the following culture-bound syndromes is this patient experiencing?

A. Amok.

B. Brain fag.

C. Dhat.

D. Koro.

E. Latah.

412 Women who experience severe nutritional deficiencies in the first trimester of pregnancy may have increased incidence of which of the following conditions in their daughters?

A. Alcohol dependence.

B. Bipolar disorder.

C. Personality disorders.

D. Post-traumatic stress disorder.

E. Schizophrenia.

409 **Answer: A.** Discrimination is where the subject has the ability to distinguish between two similar stimuli. Law of effect is one of the names given to reinforcement and it states that we retain or learn behaviour because of a satisfactory result. Stimulus generalisation occurs when a stimulus that is similar to an original stimulus elicits a conditioned response. **[AC. pp. 75–7]**

410 **Answer: B.** Age was not found to be a significant prognostic variable in this study. However, gender, marital status, acute versus gradual onset, DUP, childhood adjustment, adolescent adjustment, having close friends, street drug use and the setting (developed versus developing countries) were. **[M. pp. 617–19]**

411 **Answer: C.** Dhat is a term used in India to refer to severe anxiety and hypochondriacal concerns associated with the discharge of semen, whitish discolouration of the urine and feelings of weakness and exhaustion. Koro involves an episode of sudden and intense anxiety that the penis will recede into the body and possibly cause death. It is associated with a feeling of overwhelming panic. The patient may attempt to prevent retraction. The syndrome is reported in South and East Asia. Latah is hypersensitivity to sudden fright, often with echopraxia, echolalia, command obedience and dissociative behaviour. The syndrome has been found in many parts of the world. Brain fag is a term initially used in West Africa to refer to a condition experienced by students in response to the challenges of schooling. Symptoms include difficulties in concentrating, remembering and thinking. Amok is a dissociative episode characterised by a period of brooding followed by an outburst of violent aggressive or homicidal behaviour directed at people and objects. **[P. pp. 2286–9]**

412 **Answer: E.** An increased incidence of schizophrenia is associated with first-trimester severe nutritional deficiencies. Second and third trimester nutritional deficiencies are associated with affective disorders. **[A. p. 380; Brown AS, van Os J. Further evidence of relation between prenatal famine and major affective disorder. *Am J Psychiatry*. 2000; 157: 190–5]**

413 Which of the following is not true regarding extinction?

A. Includes a gradual loss of the conditioned response.

B. Occurs in classical conditioning when the unconditioned stimulus is omitted repeatedly.

C. Occurs in operant conditioning.

D. Refers to the ending of a psychotherapeutic relationship.

E. Results from repetition of the conditioned stimulus without reinforcement.

414 Remembering the answer when presented with a multiple-choice question of the one-best-item variety is an example of which of the following?

A. Encoding.   B. Recall.

C. Recognition.   D. Repression.

E. Retrieval.

415 Which one of the following statements regarding the epidemiology of bipolar affective disorder (BPAD) is false?

A. Comorbidity is common in BPAD.

B. Lifetime prevalence rates are considerably greater than the six-month prevalence rates.

C. The Epidemiologic Catchment Area study found a one-year prevalence rate of 1.2%.

D. The Epidemiologic Catchment Area study found that only 39% of BPAD I and BPAD II patients received outpatient psychiatric treatment in the previous year.

E. Unlike depression the prevalence rate is similar in males and females.

416 A patient with epilepsy experiences frequent seizures. He initially experiences an intense fear, followed by a period of absence, amnesia and motor activity. He is confused following the seizure. Which term best describes this seizure?

A. Petit mal.

B. Complex partial.

C. Partial seizures evolving to secondarily generalised seizures.

D. Simple partial.

E. Tonic-clonic.

413 **Answer: D.** In extinction the conditioned response tends to decrease over time when the conditioned stimulus is presented a number of times without the unconditioned stimulus. The conditioned response may partially recover after a period of rest. Extinction can take place both in classical conditioning and operant conditioning. Extinction is not a part of the psychotherapeutic relationship. **[AF. p. 33]**

414 **Answer: C.** Recognition takes place when the retrieval of the memory is facilitated by presence of a helpful stimulus. A recall takes place when a memory can be retrieved easily by an act of will. Repression is a defence mechanism in which memory is forced into the unconscious domain and encoding is a process characterised by giving an informational input a more useful form. **[AC. pp. 85–6]**

415 **Answer: B.** BPAD is a chronic recurrent condition and the lifetime and six-month prevalence rates are similar. **[E. pp. 500–22; M. p. 696]**

416 **Answer: B.** Generalised seizures involve abnormal electrical activity which is widespread in the brain and results in loss of consciousness. Partial seizures involve abnormal electrical activity in a focal area of the brain, which may or may not result in loss of consciousness. A partial seizure may evolve into a generalised seizure. Simple partial seizures usually have an abrupt onset and ending and last only a few seconds, with no loss of consciousness. Complex partial seizures are the most common type of partial seizures. They are characterised by the presences of an aura, followed by a period of absence, amnesia, loss of consciousness and motor activity. They may be accompanied by an automatism. Tonic-clonic seizures are generalised seizures involving loss of consciousness and a tonic phase during which there is sudden spasm of all the muscles of the body for several seconds. This is followed by rhythmic jerking of the limbs and head (clonic phase). Petit mal are generalised seizures characterised by loss of awareness of one's surroundings. The attack lasts a few seconds and consciousness is lost. **[A. pp. 315–16]**

417 You are a psychiatric SHO in your third year of training in an academic department and are asked by your clinical supervisor to assist on a piece of research. You decide to screen a certain population for psychiatric illness using the Present State Examination. Which of the following conditions does it have relatively good reliability for screening?

A. Alcoholism.

B. Dementia.

C. Organic conditions.

D. Personality disorders.

E. Schizophrenia.

418 A 55-year-old man is referred with psychosexual problems. He has a history of very heavy alcohol intake for the last 20 years. Which of the following would you most expect to see?

A. Increased body hair.

B. Increased breast size.

C. Increased libido.

D. Increased penis size.

E. Increased testes size.

419 According to Plutchik, there are eight primary emotions. Looking at the list below, which one is not a primary emotion?

A. Anger.

B. Anticipation.

C. Fear.

D. Love.

E. Surprise.

420 Which one of the following statements regarding the aetiology of bipolar affective disorder is false?

A. Anticipation does not occur.

B. Genetic heterogenicity is probable.

C. Several studies observed linkage with chromosome 18 markers.

D. Several studies observe X-chromosome linkage.

E. The probability that individual genes identified by linkage studies are involved in the aetiology of BPAD is not high.

417 **Answer: E.** In the screening of a given population for psychiatric illness, the Present State Examination (Wing, *et al.* 1974) has relatively good reliability in diagnosing schizophrenia. It also has relatively poor reliability for diagnosing alcoholism, personality disorders and organic conditions. **[AS. p. 307]**

418 **Answer: B.** Long-standing marked alcohol abuse can lead to gynaecomastia in men. It can also lead to a decrease in most of the other items listed. In women it can lead to vaginal dryness, breast shrinking and disturbances of menstruation. **[R. p. 341]**

419 **Answer: D:** According to Plutchik, there are eight primary emotions which are disgust, anger, anticipation, joy, acceptance, fear, surprise and sadness. Any two primary emotions can give rise to a secondary emotion: love is an example of a secondary emotion made from the primary emotions of joy and acceptance. **[G. p. 9]**

420 **Answer: A.** Anticipation implies that a disease occurs at a progressively earlier age of onset and with more severe symptoms in successive generations. It has been demonstrated in BPAD, unipolar depression, Huntington's, myotonic dystrophy and others. It is associated with trinucleotide repeats. The inheritance of BPAD is not Mendelian and genetic studies are complicated by different presentations of bipolar spectrum disorders. Chromosomes implicated with linkage studies include 4, 5, 11, 12, 18, and X. **[M. pp. 701–4]**

421 A 55-year-old patient who has been drinking alcohol heavily for over 10 years attends the service requesting information about alcohol support services. At what stage of the change cycle is this patient?

A. Action.

B. Contemplation.

C. Decision.

D. Maintenance.

E. Precontemplation.

422 A 45-year-old man with a long history of borderline personality disorder and multiple attendances at A&E departments attends your local A&E for assessment. He requests admission to the psychiatric department. Following mental state examination, you decide not to admit this man. Which of the following types of processing are you most likely using in making this decision?

A. Bottom-up processing.

B. Due process.

C. Primary process.

D. Secondary process.

E. Top-down processing.

423 Which of the following is not used in measurement of attitude?

A. Likert scales.

B. Present State Examination.

C. Questionnaires.

D. Semantic differential scales.

E. Thurstone scales.

424 A boy after watching a Harry Potter movie believes that cars can fly. According to Piaget's cognitive development theory, at which stage is he at present?

A. Sensori-motor stage

B. Pre-operational stage.

C. Concrete operational stage.

D. Formal operational stage.

E. Oral stage.

421 **Answer: C.** The cycle of change proposed by Prochaska and DiClemente, originally developed to describe the process people go through in giving up smoking, is also applied to drinking behaviour. The stages are as follows:

- Precontemplation – the person does not see any harm in their behaviour.
- Contemplation – the person is unsure whether they want to change their behaviour or not.
- Decision/Determination – they person has decided to do something and is getting ready for change.
- Action – the person has made the change.
- Maintenance – the change has been integrated into the person's life.
- Relapse – there is full return of the old behaviour.

The man in the question has decided to change and is preparing to do so by seeking support. **[S. pp. 237–8]**

422 **Answer: E.** Top-down processing is based on our knowledge and expectations. Bottom-up processing is processing based directly on the person or object in front of us. Research into psychiatrists' decision making when it comes to management of borderline personality disorder indicates that top-down processing is used more, i.e. our knowledge and expectations rather than based on the person in front of us. Primary process is a Freudian term referring to the operating system of the unconscious mind. Due process is a legal term and so a distracter. **[C. p. 296; G. p. 95]**

423 **Answer: B.** There are several ways of measuring attitudes, e.g. projective tests and questionnaires. Likert scales involve agreeing/disagreeing on a five-point scale. Thurstone scales involve a range of statements that are presented and you pick those you agree with. A semantic differential scale is a visual analogue scale with polarised adjectives separated by a line. Subjects mark their attitude between the two. The Present State Examination is an interview schedule for mental state examination and does not measure attitudes. **[AF. p. 30]**

424 **Answer: B.** The phenomenon described in this example is of magical thinking, which is characterised by an absence of recognition of the importance of the laws of nature. According to Piaget, the sensori-motor stage is from infancy to two years of age, followed by the pre-operational stage (up to seven years of age) during which children show the phenomena of magical thinking, anthropomorphic thinking and egocentrism. This stage is followed by the concrete operational stage and formal operational stage. The oral stage is a distracter in this example. **[AC. pp. 164–5]**

425 A 25-year-old man with a history of one episode of mild depression presents with a one-week episode of mildly elated mood, increased energy, talkativeness and decreased need for sleep. He is able to attend his job (salesman) and tells you that his boss commented on his new energetic approach to his work. His wife tells you that he can't sit still at home and that his libido has increased. Which one of the following is the most appropriate ICD-10 diagnosis?

A. Bipolar affective disorder.

B. Bipolar affective disorder, current episode hypomanic.

C. Hypomanic episode.

D. Mania without psychotic symptoms.

E. Recurrent depressive disorder.

426 An EEG shows high voltage slow waves all over the scalp. δ waves account for <50% of the rhythm. Sleep spindles and K complexes diminish. What stage of the sleep cycle is this EEG detecting?

A. Stage I.   B. Stage II.

C. Stage III.   D. Stage IV.

E. Wakefulness.

427 Which of the following is not part of a standard risk assessment in psychiatry?

A. Eliciting a drug history.

B. Frontal lobe function testing.

C. History of access to or knowledge of weapons.

D. Past history of compliance with treatment.

E. Past history of violence to others.

428 A 45-year-old man is noted to have nystagmus. Which of the following would most point to a potential central cause of the nystagmus?

A. Ataxic gait.

B. Marked visual impairment.

C. Nystagmus is present only when eye movements are tested very quickly.

D. Nystagmus is present only when testing the outer edges of lateral gaze.

E. Vertigo.

425 **Answer: B.** This is an episode of hypomania, with a background of depression and therefore the diagnosis is bipolar affective disorder, current episode hypomanic (F31.0). **[I. pp. 112–28]**

426 **Answer: C.** The EEG features of sleep may be summarised as follows:

- Stage I: the occipital α rhythm slowly disappears and low-voltage desynchronised slow waves (θ and δ) appear.
- Stage II: low voltages and δ and slower frequencies dominate the recording. Sleep spindles and K complexes occur.
- Stage III: high-voltage slow waves occur all over the scalp. δ waves account for <50% of the rhythm. Sleep spindles and K complexes diminish.
- Stage IV: δ waves dominate the EEG accounting for >50% of the rhythm. Sleep spindles and K complexes are absent.
- Wakefulness: characterised by the high-frequency β rhythm.

[S. p. 536]

427 **Answer: B.** Frontal lobe testing is not part of a standard risk assessment. However, if there is a suspicion regarding an organic cause, further investigation and neuropsychiatric testing may be required. Also part of a standard risk assessment are: evidence of social restlessness, mental state examination for delusions, specific threats and emotions related to violence, i.e. irritability, anger and suspiciousness. **[AF. p. 288]**

428 **Answer: A.** The causes of nystagmus can be divided into four categories. Physiological causes are normal and include situations such as items C and D. Retinal causes mainly cause pendular nystagmus (as opposed to jerk nystagmus) and include marked visual impairment. Peripheral causes include damage to the vestibular nerve or the labyrinth: thus vertigo might point to a peripheral cause. Central causes include vestibular nuclei damage and cerebellar damage: the latter of course can cause ataxia. **[AU. pp. 40–2]**

429 In your outpatient clinic you get a patient with a lot of psychiatric and personality difficulties and you decide to request a Minnesota Multiphasic Personality Inventory test. Which of the following is not a clinical scale of MMPI?

A. Body perception.

B. Hypochondriasis.

C. Hysteria.

D. Masculinity/Femininity.

E. Social introversion.

430 Concerning the aetiology of depression, which one of the following statements is false?

A. 5-HT receptor polymorphisms are associated with affective disorders.

B. Adoption studies support the genetic theory of aetiology of depression.

C. Anticipation does not occur in depression.

D. Kendler proposed that genetic factors increase the risk of onset of depression by increasing the sensitivity of individuals to depression-inducing effects of life events.

E. Twin studies support the genetic theory of aetiology of depression.

431 A 25-year-old man with schizophrenia tells you that thoughts are being taken out of his head by terrorists. He says his head goes blank after this. He believes that these terrorists are responsible for transmitting his thoughts to others, who use his words to write songs. What form of thought disorder is this man experiencing?

A. Audible thoughts.

B. Thought blocking.

C. Thought broadcasting.

D. Thought insertion.

E. Thought withdrawal.

432 Which of the following tests of intelligence does not rely on recall of information?

A. Raven's Progressive Matrices.

B. Stanford–Binet Intelligence Scale.

C. Wechsler Adult Intelligence Scale (WAIS).

D. Wechsler Intelligence Scale for Children-Revised (WISC-R).

E. Wechsler Pre-school and Primary School Intelligence Scale (WPPSI).

429 **Answer: A.** The following are the scales of MMPI: Hypochondriasis, Depression, Hysteria, Psychopathic Deviation, Masculinity/Femininity, Paranoia, Psychasthenia, Schizophrenia, Hypomania, Social Introversion. **[AE. pp. 207–8]**

430 **Answer: C.** Anticipation does occur in depression. Twin, family and adoption studies support the genetic theory of depression but environmental factors are very important too. Kendler found that genetic factors increase the risk of onset of depression by increasing the sensitivity of individuals to the depression-inducing effects of life events. 5-HT receptor polymorphisms and allelic association between the serotonin transporter gene and unipolar depression have been found. **[M. p. 704; T. p. 302]**

431 **Answer: B.** Option B is a disorder of thought form. Option A is a type of auditory hallucination. The remaining options are delusions, or disorders of thought content. Thought blocking is a form of thought disorder in which the patient experiences his chain of thoughts snapping off or stopping unexpectedly. This patient interprets this experience as a delusion of thought control. He believes that his thoughts are being taken out of his head by another agency (thought withdrawal). In an additional delusion of thought control he also believes that his thoughts are being dispersed widely out of his control (thought broadcasting). Thought insertion is a third delusion of thought control, in which the patient believes that thoughts are being inserted into his head. This is a delusional interpretation of the thought disorder. Audible thoughts, in which a patient hears their own thoughts out loud, is a form of auditory hallucination. **[D. pp. 140–1, 148–9]**

432 **Answer: A.** Raven's Progressive Matrices involves diagram completion and does not rely on recall. Hence it is less sensitive to cultural differences and can be used for people with communication difficulties. **[F. p. 41]**

433 The verbal component of the Wechsler Adult Intelligence Scale (WAIS-III) contains all the following except:

A. Arithmetic.

B. Digit span.

C. Digit symbol.

D. Information.

E. Letter number sequencing.

434 During a ward round your consultant says that one patient is using mature defence mechanisms. Of the list given below, which of the following is a mature defence mechanism?

A. Dissociation.

B. Isolation.

C. Humour.

D. Passive-aggressive behaviour.

E. Projection.

435 A 40-year-old female patient loses her job. Which one of the following factors is not thought to increase her vulnerability for developing depression?

A. Being employed away from home.

B. Being socially isolated.

C. Having three or more children under the age of 14.

D. Lack of a confiding relationship.

E. Loss of her mother before the age of 11.

436 A 55-year-old patient with a history of alcohol dependence is admitted to the hospital for alcohol detoxification. He is noted on assessment to have clouding of consciousness. On physical examination he is found to have paralysis of the external rectus muscle, paralysis of conjugate gaze, ataxia and peripheral polyneuropathy. Ophthalmoscopic examination reveals retinal haemorrhages. What vitamin deficiency is responsible for this clinical picture?

A. A.

B. B_1.

C. B_{12}

D. E.

E. K.

433 **Answer: C.** The Wechsler Adult Intelligence Scale (WAIS-III) has two scales, verbal and spatial (or performance), each of which has several sub-tests. The verbal scale includes arithmetic, comprehension, digit span, information, letter-number sequencing, similarities and vocabulary. The performance scale includes block design, digit symbol, matrix reasoning, object assembly, picture arrangement, picture completion and symbol search. **[M. p. 97]**

434 **Answer: C.** The following are considered the mature defence mechanisms:

- altruism
- anticipation
- asceticism
- humour
- sublimation
- suppression. **[K. pp. 207–8]**

435 **Answer: A.** Brown and Harris' work identified several factors as increasing women's vulnerability to depression following a life event. These are: being unemployed, having three or more children under the age of 14, lack of a confiding relationship and loss of the mother before the age of 11. Bowlby believed that being socially isolated was a vulnerability factor because of lack of necessary attachments. **[M. pp. 704–5; T. p. 99]**

436 **Answer: C.** [handwritten: B] This patient has developed Wernicke's encephalopathy as a result of vitamin B_{12} or thiamine deficiency. He is likely to be deficient in all vitamins as a result of malnutrition. **[A. p. 1105]**

437 A two-month-old infant smiles at his mother. The mother observes this and believes that the child is responding to her. At what age does social smiling begin in the infant?

A. Birth.

B. One month.

C. Two months.

D. Three months.

E. Four months.

438 A 22-year-old woman with anorexia nervosa has proximal myopathy. She complains of difficulty in brushing her hair. When asked to shrug her shoulders she can do this reasonably but cannot raise them when you push down on her shoulders with a small degree of force. What is the correct Medical Research Council Power Scale score to describe this?

A. 1

B. 2.

C. 3

D. 4.

E. 5.

439 Which of the following can obstruct proper history taking?

A. Acknowledging emotions.

B. Encouragement.

C. Judgemental views.

D. Neutral facial expression.

E. Reassurance.

440 Which one of the following statements regarding the endocrine dysfunction model of aetiology of depression is false?

A. Administering cortisol synthesis-inhibiting chemicals may be effective for treating depression.

B. Hypercortisolaemia is found in approximately half of cases of depression.

C. Non-suppression of the dexamethasone suppression test (DST) is found in 60–70% of depressed (melancholic) patients.

D. The non-suppression of the DST is not diagnostic of depression.

E. There is persistent atrophy of the adrenal glands.

437 **Answer: D.** Smiling in the infant may observed soon after birth. Any pleasing stimulus may elicit a smile from birth onwards; social smiling begins from three months. **[AP. p. 153]**

438 **Answer: C.** The MRC scale for power is graded from 0 to 5. A score of 3 indicates that the patient has active movement of the muscle group against gravity but not against resistance from the examiner. **[AU. pp. 51–2]**

439 **Answer: C.** Judgemental views, minimisation, premature advice, compound questions and trapping the patient in his or her own words can obstruct proper history taking. **[K. p. 47]**

440 **Answer: E.** The adrenal glands are hypertrophied in depression. **[T. pp. 278–9; M. pp. 714–15]**

441 A 44-year-old man is referred for assessment by his GP who reports that he has been complaining of memory loss following a road traffic accident. Which of the following findings would suggest that this man is malingering?

A. Dense anterograde amnesia.

B. Loss of consciousness at the time of the accident.

C. Performance worse than chance level on neuropsychological testing.

D. Perseveration.

E. Retrograde amnesia.

442 A four-year-old child exhibits a similar response to a primate when a reward comes from pressing a lever to which of the schedules described below?

A. Constant interval.

B. Fixed interval.

C. Fixed ratio.

D. Variable interval.

E. Variable ratio.

443 The sick role as defined by Parsons includes all of the following except:

A. Abnormal illness behaviour.

B. Exemption from normal social role responsibilities.

C. Obligation to seek and cooperate with treatment.

D. The expectation of a desire to get well.

E. The right to expect help and care.

444 You are seeing Albert, a 24-year-old man, in an outpatient clinic. He is quite worried about a single episode of blackout where he became violent after drinking alcohol for the first time. He tells you that he can remember sleeping for a prolonged period of time. Which of the following is the best description of Albert's condition?

A. Automatism.

B. Clouding of consciousness.

C. Delirium tremens.

D. *Mania à potu.*

E. Twilight state.

441 **Answer: C.** The diagnosis of malingering is made when the features of the presentation and history are atypical for an amnestic disorder. The patient may feign amnesia in preparation for legal proceedings. On neuropsychological testing a pattern of performance that is worse than chance or guessing suggests manipulation of the results for deliberate failure. Densely amnestic patients score at least at a chance level of 50% accuracy simply by guessing. Malingering patients may purposely avoid the correct response and score below chance. On tests of progressive difficulty the malingering patient might perform poorly even on the easier tasks and may not demonstrate the graduated decrements in performance of an amnestic patient. The remaining options are suggestive of a true amnesia. **[A. p. 1105]**

442 **Answer: B.** Children up to age five years show similar response as animals to fixed-interval schedules in which a reward comes from pressing a particular lever. **[AP. pp. 31–2]**

443 **Answer: A.** Abnormal illness behaviour is associated with Pilowsky. It refers to maladaptive ways of responding to one's own health status despite adequate advice and management by health professionals. **[E. p. 822; B. p. 719]**

444 **Answer: D.** *Mania à potu* is a specific type of twilight state and is characterised by four components:

- consumption of a variable quantity of alcohol
- senseless violent behaviour
- prolonged sleep after the violent act
- total or partial amnesia.

It is differentiated from delirium, which is a symptom of withdrawal while *mania à potu* occurs in intoxicated conditions. Another name for *mania à potu* is pathological intoxication. **[D. pp. 34–5]**

445 Sleep disturbance is common in depression. Which one of the following statements is false?

   A. Depressed patients show super-sensitivity to the REM sleep effects of cholinergic agonists.

   B. REM latency is decreased.

   C. Sleep deprivation may give a transient elevation of mood.

   D. Total slow-wave sleep is increased.

   E. Tricyclic antidepressants suppress REM sleep.

446 A man who believes in the rights of the disabled finds that there is no parking space beside his workplace. It is raining heavily and he is late for an important meeting. There are two parking spaces for the disabled available. He parks in a disabled parking space. Which of the following factors will decrease his cognitive dissonance?

   A. A sign requesting that drivers refrain from using the disabled parking spaces.

   B. Deciding that disabled parking spaces discriminate against drivers without a disability.

   C. The approach of a traffic warden.

   D. The knowledge that there are parking spaces five minutes' walk away.

   E. The knowledge that two of his co-workers are disabled.

447 The effect of new learning can make it more difficult to retrieve old information. What is this phenomenon called?

   A. Proactive interference.   **B.** Selective attention.

   C. State-dependent learning.   **D.** Retroactive interference.

   E. Retrograde amnesia.

448 A 53-year-old man is asked to stand with his feet together. He stands steady during this. He is then asked to close his eyes. He falls over within a couple of seconds. Which of the following best describes this?

   A. Negative Weber's test.   **B.** Positive Babinski response.

   C. Positive Kernig's sign.   **D.** Positive Rinne's test.

   E. Positive Romberg's test.

445 **Answer: D.** Slow-wave sleep and REM latency are decreased in depression whereas REM duration is increased. Cholinergics are 'pro-REM sleep' and depressed patients are super-sensitive to them. Anticholinergics (e.g. tricyclic antidepressants) are REM suppressors. Short-term sleep deprivation can give a transient rise in mood. **[T. p. 282; M. p. 715]**

446 **Answer: B.** Cognitive dissonance theory, proposed by Festinger in 1957, suggests that individuals strive for consistency in their attitudes, with discomfort or dissonance arising if two cognitions are held that are inconsistent. Dissonance is increased by low pressure to comply, increased choice of options, awareness of responsibility for consequences and expectation of unpleasant consequences of behaviour towards others. Dissonance is decreased by changing behaviour, dismissing information and adding new cognitions. This man decreases his dissonance by changing his attitudes towards the rights of the disabled. **[S. p. 93]**

447 **Answer: D.** There are two main types of interference: proactive inhibition and retroactive interference. Retroactive interference is the deleterious effect of new learning upon retrieval of old information. Proactive interference is the opposite. **[AP. p. 59]**

448 **Answer: E.** It indicates difficulties in the man's proprioception. Cerebellar disease may be indicated if the man sways back and forth when his eyes were closed. **[AU. p. 67]**

449 A patient who talks a lot about irrelevant things before reaching the final point of discussion is showing which of the following?

A. Circumstantiality.

B. Condensation.

C. Flight of ideas.

D. Incoherence.

E. Tangentiality.

450 Polysomnography was performed on a young man who complained of fatigue. You notice frequent 0.5 second bursts of 12–14 Hertz waves on the EEG. Which of the following sleep stages are you most likely to be observing?

A. REM sleep.

B. Stage I Non-REM sleep.

C. Stage II Non-REM sleep.

D. Stage III Non-REM sleep.

E. Stage IV Non-REM sleep.

451 A 40-year-old patient with a history of alcohol dependence syndrome is currently abstinent from alcohol. He reports that he feels ready to return to work. Which of the following features of this man's plans for employment would least concern you?

A. Autonomous working.

B. Job mobility.

C. Office environment.

D. Sale of alcohol.

E. Spending much time away from home.

452 A baby of nine months knows that when her mother hides her toy, the toy although no longer visible still exists. Which term best describes this phenomenon?

A. Good enough mother.

B. Object permanence.

C. Projective identification.

D. Potential space.

E. Transitional object.

449 **Answer: A.** Circumstantiality is indirect speech that is delayed in reaching the point but eventually gets there: it is characterised by over-inclusion of details. In tangentiality the speaker never gets from the start to the desired goal. **[K. p. 283]**

450 **Answer: C.** These are sleep spindles and are characteristic of stage II Non-REM sleep. Stages III and IV are known as slow-wave sleep and the relative amount of these decreases with age. **[P. p. 281]**

451 **Answer: C.** The factors which increase the risk of relapse in the work environment are job mobility, an absence of the restraining structure of home/regular workplace, the absence of supervision at work and the ready availability of alcohol. **[H. p. 121]**

452 **Answer: B.** By eight months infants begin to attain the concept of object permanence. They begin to understand the concept that objects still exist although they may not be visible to the infant. A transitional object is used by an infant for anxiety reduction and self-soothing. The potential space is an area of experiencing identified as existing between the baby and the object. A good enough mother is a mother who responds to her baby and meets their needs in an optimal zone of frustration and satisfaction. Potential space, good enough mother, and transitional object are all terms described by Winnicott. **[AP. p. 156; G. p. 102]**

453 When you look up a new telephone number and hold on to it long enough to dial, one of the following is not correct:

A. The duration of recall can be extended by rehearsing.

B. The information can be held up to 15 to 30 seconds.

C. The number of digits that can be held can be increased by chunking.

D. This type of memory can be assessed by digit repetition.

E. This type of memory is also known as semantic memory.

454 A patient with schizophrenia mentioned to a staff nurse that he can hear his parents talking about him in the train station (located two miles away). Which of the following psychopathological terms best describes this?

A. Extracampine hallucination.

B. Functional hallucination.

C. Reflex hallucination.

D. Second-person auditory hallucination.

E. Third-person auditory hallucination.

455 A man lying on the grass and staring at the sky sees the figure of the devil's face in the shape of the clouds. Which of the following best describes this?

A. Anthropomorphism.

B. Extracampine visual hallucination.

C. Mirage.

D. Pareidolia.

E. Visual hallucination.

456 A patient with bipolar affective disorder on lithium therapy complains of sudden onset of tremor. His speech is slurred at interview and his gait is unsteady. His serum lithium is 2.0 mmol/L. Which of the following is most likely to have contributed to the development of lithium toxicity?

A. Alcohol.

B. Caffeine.

C. Frusemide.

D. Lamotrigine.

E. Warfarin.

453 **Answer: E.** This refers to working memory, which is also known as short-term, immediate, primary or buffer memory. Working memory holds 7+2 bits of information for up to 15–30 seconds. The number of bits can be increased by chunking. The period can be extended by rehearsing. We use working memory when looking up a new telephone number and holding on to it long enough to dial. Working memory may be assessed by digit repetition or digit reversal. Semantic memory is not a synonym: it is the knowledge of facts, concepts and language etc. **[E. p. 387; M. p. 271]**

454 **Answer: A.** Extracampine hallucinations are experienced outside the limits of the sensory field. In functional hallucinations an external stimulus is necessary to provoke hallucinations. In reflex hallucinations a stimulus in one sensory modality produces hallucinations in another. **[D. p. 96]**

455 **Answer: D.** This describes pareidolia which occurs in a considerable proportion of normal people and can also be provoked by illicit drugs. **[T. p. 84]**

456 **Answer: C.** Thiazide diuretics reduce the renal clearance of lithium and levels can rise within a few days. Excessive caffeine can cause a decrease in lithium levels. A rapid decrease in caffeine intake can result in lithium toxicity. Alcohol may result in a slight increase (about 12%) in peak lithium levels. There is no documented interaction between lithium and lamotrigine or warfarin. **[X. pp. 302–6]**

457 A married father of three children has alcohol dependence syndrome. His wife describes a strained marital relationship as a result of his drinking. He enjoys a close relationship with his eldest daughter. What term describes this dynamic in the family relationship?

A. Rejection.

B. Repression.

C. Reversal into the opposite.

D. Splitting.

E. Triangulation.

458 Which of the following is not a stage in Kohlberg's Stage Theory of Moral Development?

A. Instrumental relativist orientation.

B. 'Good-boy/nice-girl' orientation.

C. Maintaining the social order orientation.

D. Punishment and obedience orientation.

E. Self-actualisation orientation.

459 A patient who is an inpatient in your ward with the diagnosis of paranoid schizophrenia says that all the nursing staff are aliens. He never had this belief before but since he came to hospital the patient in the bed next to him, with whom he gets on very well, has given him this idea. In terms of psychopathology, which of the following is the best description of this condition?

A. *Folie à deux.*

B. *Folie communiquée.*

C. *Folie imposée.*

D. *Folie induite.*

E. *Folie simultanée.*

460 Clozapine is indicted for treatment resistance in schizophrenia. Which one of the following is associated with clozapine?

A. $5HT_2$ agonism.

B. Impotence secondary to hyperprolactinaemia.

C. Nocturnal enuresis.

D. Strong D_2 receptor antagonism.

E. Tardive dyskinesia.

457 **Answer: E.** *Triangulation*, a type of dysfunctional familial structural pattern, may be used to solve a serious problem within the family unit. A strong father–daughter alliance may prevent the father from leaving the family unit. A to D are Freudian defence mechanisms. **[AP. p. 271]**

458 **Answer: E.** Options D and A (stages 1 and 2 respectively) are part of Kohlberg's Level 1: *Preconventional Morality*. Items B and C likewise are stages 3 and 4 of Level 2: *Conventional Morality*. Level 3: *Postconventional Morality* is comprised of stage 5: social contract-legalistic orientation and stage 6: universal principles orientation. *Self-actualisation* is a term from Maslow's hierarchy of needs. **[O. pp. 512–13]**

459 **Answer: D.** These are all examples of communicated psychotic symptoms, broadly described as *folie à deux*, which has four further subdivisions. In *folie imposée* and *communiquée* delusional ideas are communicated to people without mental illness, while in *folie induite* a person who is already psychotic adds the delusion of a person close to him to his own psychotic beliefs. **[D. pp. 124–5]**

460 **Answer: C.** Clozapine is not thought to cause tardive dyskinesia or hyperprolactinaemia. This may be secondary to its $5HT_2$ blockade and its low D_2 blockade. It can cause nocturnal enuresis. **[V. pp. 70–1; Z. p. 73]**

461 A 54-year-old woman is due to have electroconvulsive therapy for the treatment of a severe depressive episode. She is reluctant as she has heard that it can cause severe memory problems. What type of memory difficulty is this patient most likely to experience?

A. Immediate memory impairment.

B. Long-term permanent anterograde amnesia.

C. Retrograde amnesia for remote events.

D. Short-term anterograde amnesia.

E. Short-term retrograde amnesia.

462 A 25-year-old man, whose father has alcohol dependence syndrome, asks you about his risk of becoming an alcoholic. Which of the following factors does not contribute to the development of alcohol dependence syndrome?

A. Alcoholic personality.

B. Modelling.

C. Occupation-related factors.

D. Operant conditioning.

E. Peer-group pressures.

463 A 20-year-old woman reports having frequent dreams when asleep. Which one of the following mechanisms is unlikely to be involved in her dream work?

A. Condensation.

B. Displacement.

C. Repression.

D. Secondary revision.

E. Symbolic representation.

464 A person has disorder of sexual preference. According to ICD-10 which of the following is therefore not a possible diagnosis?

A. Fetishism.

B. Voyeurism.

C. Paedophilia.

D. Transsexualism.

E. Sadomasochism.

461 **Answer: D.** Most patients will experience some degree of anterograde amnesia, particularly if the patient is confused after the treatment. Some patients will have difficulty retaining new learning for a few days or even weeks after a course of ECT. This impairment, while common, is short lived. A smaller number of patients will experience a retrograde amnesia for events leading up to and during a course of ECT. Some patients will report holes or gaps in their memory extending back several years. The issue of long-term permanent anterograde amnesia is unresolved but is complained of only by a minority. Immediate memory refers to the sensory store in which information is held for less than a second in the form in which it was perceived. This level is not usually affected in organic memory disorders. **[A. pp. 894–6; D. p. 49]**

462 **Answer: A.** There is no evidence for an alcohol personality. Modelling is a possible explanation for increased family risk of alcohol dependence; adoption studies do not support this. Operant conditioning views reinforcement of drinking as coming from wishing to avoid withdrawal symptoms. Higher-risk occupations, i.e. brewers, publicans etc., and peer-group pressure are regularly referred to by journalists (another group at high risk to develop alcohol dependence). **[H. p. 123]**

463 **Answer: C.** Unacceptable content in dreams was thought by Freud to undergo changes that would prevent processing of the material from disturbing sleep. Condensation, displacement, symbolic representation and secondary revision are mechanisms of dream work. Repression is a defence mechanism. **[E. pp. 570–1]**

464 **Answer: D.** Transsexualism is a disorder of gender identity while all the other disorders are the disorders of sexual preference. Other disorders of sexual preference are: fetishistic-transvestism, exhibitionism and multiple disorders of sexual preference. **[D. pp. 245–51]**

465 A 22-year-old female patient is prescribed the oral contraceptive pill (OCP) by her GP. Which one of the following concurrently administered medications is least likely to render the OCP ineffective?

A. Carbamazepine.

B. Oxcarbazepine.

C. St John's wort.

D. Topiramate.

E. Valproate.

466 A patient is admitted to a psychiatric hospital as a voluntary patient. During his admission he tells his doctor that he no longer wishes to take medication. His doctor tells him that if he does not take medication his status will be changed to involuntary and he will be given medication by force. What ethical principle has this doctor most transgressed?

A. Autonomy.

B. Beneficence.

C. Confidentiality.

D. Justice.

E. Nonmaleficence.

467 While assessing a 50-year-old patient with a long history of schizophrenia, you note that he has marked trunk movements along with occasional tongue movements. What is the most likely diagnosis in this case?

A. Akathisia.

B. Mannerism.

C. Stereotypy.

D. Torticollis.

E. Tardive dyskinesia.

468 Choose the most correct statement regarding the pharmacology of sertindole:

A. It blocks adrenergic α_1 receptors.

B. It blocks histamine H_1 receptors.

C. It does not block $5HT_{2A}$ receptors.

D. It is a significant D_1 receptor blocker.

E. It is a significant D_4 receptor blocker.

465 **Answer: E.** Valproate does not clinically affect the metabolism of the OCP. The other medications are all used for the treatment of affective disorders. [**www.uspharmacist.com/index.asp?show=article&page=8_1193. htm**]

466 **Answer: A.** The four main ethical principles of medical treatment are as follows:

- Autonomy: respecting the freedom of the patient to make choices regarding their treatment.
- Beneficence: placing the benefit to the patient at the forefront of clinical practice.
- Nonmaleficence: doing no harm.
- Justice: this refers to both individual and social justice.

This doctor has adopted a coercive approach to treatment. While one might argue that this does harm to the patient, and certainly to the therapeutic relationship, it most clearly compromises the patient's autonomy. [**AJ. pp. 41–4**]

467 **Answer: E.** Tardive dyskinesia is a syndrome of involuntary movements developing in the course of long-term exposure to antipsychotics. Akathisia is a subjective restlessness, associated with an urge to move a part or all of the body. Torticollis is characterised by involuntary tonic contractions or intermittent spasms of neck muscles and can occur in tardive dyskinesia. A stereotypy is a spontaneous repetitive movement that is not goal directed. [**A. pp. 93–5, F. p. 89**]

468 **Answer: A.** Sertindole may cause less weight gain than other antipsychotics and has low incidence of EPSE but some concerns remain regarding QTc prolongation (as with other antipsychotics). It produces blockade of a number of receptors: D_2, D_3, $5HT_{2A}$, $5HT_{2c}$, $5HT_6$, $5HT_7$ and α_1 adrenergic receptors. [**Z. pp. 84–5**]

469 A patient says that he can hear colours. In psychopathological terminology which of the following best describes this condition?

A. Abnormal energy.

B. Functional hallucination.

C. Extracampine hallucination.

D. Reflex hallucination.

E. Synaesthesia.

470 Which one of the following descriptions is not a characteristic of schizoid personality disorder?

A. Aloofness.

B. Excessive preoccupation with fantasy.

C. Odd behaviour.

D. Quasi-psychotic episodes.

E. Social withdrawal.

471 A 35-year-old male patient with schizophrenia and a history of violence when unwell reports that he has stopped taking his medication as he was experiencing intolerable side-effects. He reports that he has been thinking about killing his psychiatrist whom he blames for the breakdown of his marriage. He also expresses a number of delusional beliefs about his ex-wife's fidelity. A decision is taken to admit the man as an involuntary patient. Which of the following best represents the ethical tension that this scenario presents?

A. Autonomy versus Beneficence.

B. Autonomy versus Nonmaleficence.

C. Beneficence versus Justice.

D. Beneficence versus Nonmaleficence.

E. Nonmaleficence versus Justice.

472 A four-year-old boy says proudly: 'I'm a boy!' His aunt teases him to put on his sister's dress. He runs away, saying, 'No! I don't want to be a girl!' What stage of Kohlberg's cognitive-developmental theory has he attained?

A. Basic gender identity.

B. Gender consistency.

C. Gender identity.

D. Gender role.

E. Gender stability.

469 **Answer: E.** Synaesthesia is the experience of a stimulus in one sense modality producing an experience in another sensory modality. A stimulus in one sensory modality producing a hallucination in another is called a reflex hallucination. In functional hallucinations, an external stimulus is necessary to provoke the hallucinations. In extracampine hallucinations, the hallucinations are experienced outside the limits of the sensory field. Abnormal energy is a distracter in this example. **[D. p. 27]**

470 **Answer: D.** This is more suggestive of schizotypal disorder than schizoid personality disorder. However, ICD-10 recommends not using the diagnosis of schizotypal disorder because of its unclear demarcation from schizoid personality disorder and schizophrenia. **[I. pp. 95, 203]**

471 **Answer: A.** The four main ethical principles of medical treatment are as follows.

- Autonomy: respecting the freedom of the patient to make choices regarding their treatment.
- Beneficence: placing the benefit to the patient at the forefront of clinical practice.
- Nonmaleficence: doing no harm.
- Justice: this refers to both individual and social justice.

In this scenario the patient's right to make choices about his treatment is in conflict with the doctor's obligation to do good for the patient. Given the stated intent to harm a specified person, the psychiatrist is most likely to treat the patient against his will, overruling his autonomy. This scenario might also be represented by a tension between autonomy and justice, considering the doctor's duty to protect third parties under certain circumstances. **[AJ. pp. 41–4]**

472 **Answer: A.** According to Kohlberg's cognitive-developmental theory basic gender identity is attained at age two to five years. In this case the child knows he is a boy but believes that it would be possible to change sex by certain actions, e.g. wearing clothes of the opposite sex. Gender stability occurs between five and six years, i.e. an awareness that gender is stable over time, but less certain that sex remains the same across different situations. Gender consistency comes around six to seven years and older, i.e. gender is stable across time and across situations. **[C. pp. 196–7]**

473 Which of the following is involved in the psychoanalytic theories of OCD?

A. All items below are involved.

B. Isolation.

C. Magical undoing.

D. Reaction formation.

E. Regression from Oedipal to anal phase.

474 Your consultant hasn't kept up to date with recent advances in psychiatric research. He asks you about something he has just heard about: Schneiderian first-rank symptoms of schizophrenia. Look at the list given below and tell him which of the following is not a first-rank symptom.

A. Audible thoughts.   B. Delusional percept.

C. Persecutory delusion.   D. Somatic passivity.

E. Thought broadcasting.

475 A man has a head injury following which his personality changes from a mild retiring disposition to a reckless aggressive one. He also develops urinary incontinence. Which one of the following brain structures is most likely to be affected?

A. Amygdalas (bilaterally).   B. Cerebellum.

C. Frontal lobe.   D. Hippocampus.

E. Temporal lobe.

476 A 36-year-old man with an episode of severe depression, unresponsive to antidepressant therapy, is undergoing a course of ECT. On his first treatment, despite two applications of an electrical stimulus, the fit is of sub-maximal duration. Which of the following medications is most likely to be causing the difficulty?

A. Chlorpromazine.   B. Clomipramine.

C. Diazepam.   D. Lithium.

E. Phenelzine.

473 **Answer: A.** Psychoanalytic theories of OCD include regression from the Oedipal to anal phase and the following defence mechanisms: isolation, magical undoing and reaction formation. OCD develops when patients fail to contain the anxiety produced by the unconscious aggressive or sexual impulses. **[E. p. 1472; M. p. 826; B. p. 661]**

474 **Answer: C.** Persecutory delusions are not part of Schneiderian first-rank symptoms. The other first-rank symptoms are: voices arguing or discussing, voices commenting on the patient's actions, thought insertion, thought withdrawal, and passivity of affect, impulse and volition. **[D. p. 164]**

475 **Answer: C.** Other changes found in frontal lobe lesions include: perseveration, psychomotor retardation, impaired concentration and attention and anosmia. **[L. p. 17; AW. pp. 60–1]**

476 **Answer: C.** Benzodiazepines are likely to raise the seizure threshold, reduce seizure duration and increase the number of treatments needed. Lithium used with ECT is reported to result in severe memory difficulties, neurological difficulties and a reduced antidepressant effect. Because of the additional potential for ECT to result in lithium toxicity, this combination should be used only with very clear indications. MAOIs are normally contra-indicated with anaesthetics as they can interact with opiates, but there is thought to be no significant problem with ECT itself. Tricyclics and ECT combined are thought to produce few difficulties, although the combinations with anaesthetic agents may enhance the risk of cardiac arrhythmias and hypotension. Antipsychotics lower the seizure threshold and would be expected to lead to seizures at lower ECT doses. **[X. pp. 158–60]**

477 You are a first-year SHO in psychiatry and are asked by your consultant to reduce the typical antipsychotic depot of a patient with schizophrenia who has been well for several years. Which of the following steps is not part of your management plan?

A. Decrements no more frequent than every three months.

B. Discontinuation should be seen as an end point in the process.

C. Dose should be reduced by no more than one third at a time.

D. Interval between injections should be increased up to four weeks, before reduction in dose.

E. Oral antipsychotics should be continued while depot is reduced.

478 A business has a crucial order to fulfil in the next two days. The manager, however, quits and the staff is in a panic without effective leadership. Which of the following leadership styles would be best suited to get the business through the next couple of days?

A. Autocratic.   B. Charismatic.

C. Coercive.   D. Democratic.

E. *Laissez-faire.*

479 Albert never asks any questions in the class session because he thinks that he may make a mistake and all the class will laugh at him. In terms of cognitive theory, Albert's thinking will best be described as which?

A. Catastrophising.   B. Dichotomous thinking.

C. Excessive responsibility.   D. Over-generalisation.

E. Selective abstraction.

480 Which of the following is not a cerebellar sign?

A. Dysdiadochokinesis.   B. Intention tremor.

C. Past pointing.   D. Romberg's sign.

E. Spastic gait.

477 **Answer: E.** Oral antipsychotics should be stopped prior to reduction in depot medication. Other steps in the reduction of depot are as per the Maudsley guidelines. **[V. p. 49]**

478 **Answer: A.** While democratic leadership can lead to overall increased productivity, the urgency of the situation calls for an autocratic style. Since the staff is panicking, leaving them to it as in *laissez-faire* is not much of an option. Coercive social power comes from being able to punish subjects: it is not a leadership style. **[R. p. 53]**

479 **Answer: A.** Catastrophising is a thinking style with the worse scenario being kept in mind. In over-generalisation, a scenario of one situation is generalised to every case. Selective abstraction is giving attention to the worst performances. Similarly, excessive responsibility is taking responsibility for all the bad things. Dichotomous thinking is a thinking style in which everything is considered either one extreme or the other. **[AD. p. 958]**

480 **Answer: E.** The associated gait with cerebellar lesions is ataxic. **[T. pp. 18–19; AY. pp. 55–60]**

481 Which of the following disorders typically has the oldest age at onset?

A. Anorexia nervosa.

B. Asperger's syndrome.

C. Gilles de la Tourette syndrome.

D. Obsessive compulsive disorder.

E. Social phobia.

482 A 25-year-old man attends your psychiatric clinic for assessment. He was the driver of a car when a friend, a backseat passenger, died in a car accident. Since then he feels low in mood, avoids driving, and has begun to drink more heavily. He drinks on average 6 units of alcohol two nights per week since the accident. Prior to this he drank 2 units two nights per week. What is the most likely ICD-10 diagnosis in this case?

A. Acute stress reaction.

B. Adjustment disorder – brief depressive reaction.

C. Mental and behavioural disorders due to the use of alcohol – harmful use.

D. Mental and behavioural disorders due to the use of alcohol – dependence syndrome.

E. Post-traumatic stress disorder.

483 Which of the following conditions is unlikely to cause perseveration?

A. Clouding of consciousness.

B. Frontal lobe disorders.

C. Memory impairment.

D. Obsessive compulsive disorder.

E. Schizophrenia.

484 You are doing cognitive behaviour therapy with a patient. Which of the following will not be among the techniques you will use?

A. Circular questioning.

B. Identifying maladaptive assumptions.

C. Flooding.

D. Testing automatic thoughts.

E. Thought stopping.

481 **Answer: D.** The mean age of onset for obsessive compulsive disorder is 20 years. Social phobia typically begins to develop after puberty. The mean age of onset of Gilles de la Tourette syndrome is seven years. Features of Asperger's syndrome are commonly noted from the age of three or earlier. The majority of females with anorexia nervosa have onset within five years of menarche **[H. pp. 68, 75, 93, 277, 287]**

482 **Answer: E.** Using ICD-10 an acute stress reaction is outruled due to the timeframe: two or three days after the accident symptoms should resolve. Post-traumatic stress disorder is a better fit for this clinical scenario than adjustment disorder – brief depressive reaction, because the duration of the depressive symptoms are longer than one month. His alcohol intake does not meet criteria for alcohol dependence syndrome. His intake of alcohol is also below the recommended Royal College of Physicians drinking limits and, with the information given here, harmful use is a less likely diagnosis. **[I. pp. 74–6, 146–50]**

483 **Answer: D.** Perseveration occurs when an act, phrase or thought is repeated after the proper time for it has passed. A response that was appropriate in one situation is given inappropriately in other situations. It is thought to be a disorder of the continuity of thought. Perseveration occurs in schizophrenia, frontal lobe disorders, memory impairment and clouding of consciousness: it does not occur in obsessive compulsive disorder. **[E. p. 223; M. p. 63; D. p. 54]**

484 **Answer: A.** Circular questioning is a technique used in family therapy. All other techniques are either cognitive or behavioural parts of cognitive behaviour therapy. Automatic thoughts are often negative in depression and are identified and tested with the patient. Flooding is a technique which is used in phobias in order to reduce the fear related to a particular situation. Thought stopping is another technique used in obsessive compulsive behaviour. **[AD. pp. 957–8]**

485 Which one of the following is thought to be associated with Alzheimer's dementia aetiology?

A. α-Amyloid plaques.

B. Increased acetylcholine.

C. Increased acetylcholinesterase.

D. Lewy bodies.

E. Neurofibrillary tangles made of hypophosphorylated tau protein.

486 A baby and his carer enter an unfamiliar room. A stranger enters and the carer leaves. The baby's play decreases and he appears upset. When the carer returns he greets her, stays close to her and begins to re-explore. According to Ainsworth what type of attachment is this baby displaying?

A. Autonomous.

B. Disorganised.

C. Insecure-ambivalent.

D. Insecure-avoidant.

E. Secure attachment.

487 A 32-year-old woman is grieving for her husband who died in a road traffic accident. You are asked to assess her by her GP. Which of the following is not a stage of normal bereavement?

A. Alarm.

B. Depression.

C. Numbness.

D. Pining for the deceased.

E. Psychomotor retardation.

488 Regarding DSM-IV criteria for personality disorder, select the most incorrect pairing:

A. Avoidant personality disorder – reluctant to take risks.

B. Borderline personality disorder – identity disturbance.

C. Dissocial personality disorder – lack of remorse.

D. Histrionic personality disorder – suggestibility.

E. Schizotypal personality disorder – excessive social anxiety.

485 **Answer: D.** β-Amyloid plaques, decreased acetylcholinesterase, choline acetyl transferase and acetylcholine, and neurofibrillary tangles made of *hyperphosphorylated* tau protein are associated with Alzheimer's dementia aetiology. **[L. p. 444; M. pp. 392–3]**

486 **Answer: E.** 60–70% of infants show secure attachment. Insecure-avoidant infants do not appear upset as the mother leaves. On her return they stay close to her but avoid her if picked up (20%). Infants with an insecure-ambivalent attachment appear upset when left, but are ambivalent on her return, reaching out but pushing her away at the same time (10%). Infants in the disorganised attachment category lack consistency in their behaviour (10–15%). Autonomous is a form of adult attachment which has been linked to childhood secure attachment. **[S. p. 66]**

487 **Answer: E.** Marked psychomotor retardation may be used to diagnose a depressive disorder from a bereavement reaction, as can marked guilt feelings, marked worthlessness and marked psychosocial functional impairment. Parkes described five stages of bereavement: alarm, numbness, pining for the deceased, depression, recovery and reorganisation. **[R. pp. 82–3]**

488 **Answer: C.** While all the criteria and personality disorder pairings are correct, DSM-IV of course uses the term 'antisocial' whereas ICD-10 uses 'dissocial'. **[R. pp. 471–4]**

489 A patient is brought to you with a psychotic illness characterised by third-person auditory hallucinations. Which of the following is not indicative of good insight?

A. He believes he is physically unwell.

B. He believes he needs medication.

C. He believes he suffers from schizophrenia.

D. He believes his symptoms are abnormal.

E. He is willing to accept advice.

490 Which one of the following is false concerning Korsakoff's syndrome?

A. Digit span test is intact.

B. In Victor's study 17% died in the acute phase.

C. It can be caused by thiamine deficiency.

D. It may follow Wernicke's encephalopathy.

E. Left hippocampal destruction is a cause.

491 A 45-year-old patient with schizophrenia is unemployed and lives with his mother. Attempts have been made to engage him in an occupational therapy programme, but he shows poor motivation. He was last hospitalised about two years ago when he had persecutory delusions, delusions of reference and second- and third-party auditory hallucinations. More recently he appears to harbour the same delusions but is not preoccupied by them. He reports that he occasionally hears voices but they don't bother him. According to DSM-IV what type of schizophrenia does this man have?

A. Catatonic.

B. Disorganised.

C. Paranoid.

D. Residual.

E. Undifferentiated.

492 A 76-year-old man living alone believes that one year ago his neighbour started putting a poison gas into his house through the heating system. This man has no medical or psychiatric history of note. Mental state examination is otherwise unremarkable. What is the most likely diagnosis in this case?

A. Delusional disorder.

B. Dementia in Alzheimer's disease.

C. Paranoid schizophrenia.

D. Paranoid personality disorder.

E. Organic delusional disorder.

489 **Answer: A.** Believing that the symptoms and the illness are psychiatric problems is a part of good insight. If somebody believed that psychotic symptoms are because of a medical illness, it is not full insight. **[AB. p. 70]**

490 **Answer: E.** Bilateral hippocampal destruction is required. **[T. p. 420]**

491 **Answer: D.** Residual schizophrenia involves an absence of prominent delusions, hallucinations, disorganised speech or grossly disorganised or catatonic behaviour. There is continuing evidence of disturbance with negative symptoms or two or more positive symptoms present in attenuated form. In disorganised schizophrenia, disorganised speech, disorganised behaviour and a flat or inappropriate affect are prominent. Catatonic schizophrenia is characterised by at least two of the following: motor immobility, excessive motor activity, extreme negativism, peculiarities of voluntary movement, or echolalia or echopraxia. Paranoid schizophrenia involves a preoccupation with one or more delusions or frequent auditory hallucinations. In undifferentiated schizophrenia the patient meets the core criteria for schizophrenia but criteria for the other subtypes are not met. **[AH. pp. 155–7]**

492 **Answer: A.** Delusional disorder is the most likely diagnosis. With no medical or past psychiatric history organic causes and dementia are outruled. Paranoid personality involves long-standing beliefs; this man has a one-year history only. The main differential is paranoid schizophrenia; in this case mental state examination revealed no other findings e.g. negative symptoms, hallucination or memory problems. This points to delusional disorder being the most likely diagnosis. **[I. pp. 62, 99–100, 202–3]**

493 When you see patients in the psychiatric ward, which of the following is not applicable to the interview technique?

A. Restitution.

B. Recapitulation.

C. Reframing.

D. Reattribution.

E. Relaxation.

494 If a patient has just negative symptoms of schizophrenia, then from the list given below, which is the most unlikely symptom to be present?

A. Abulia.

B. Alogia.

C. Apathy.

D. Avolition.

E. Neologism.

495 High levels of expressed emotion have been found to increase the risk of schizophrenic relapse. Which of the following pairs of researchers is associated with this finding?

A. Brown and Birley.

B. Brown and Harris.

C. Holmes and Rahe.

D. Vaughan and Leff.

E. Wing and Brown.

496 A 40-year-old man is referred for assessment. While taking his history you note that he expresses a lot of anger towards his parents and is preoccupied with events from his childhood. According to Main, which form of adult attachment is this man likely to display?

A. Autonomous.

B. Dismissing.

C. Disorganised.

D. Preoccupied.

E. Unresolved.

493 **Answer: E.** Restitution, which is restoring something or compensation, is useful when interviewing patients. Recapitulating, reframing, reattribution and rephrasing are other techniques used when interviewing patients. Relaxation is not an interview technique. **[A. p. 237]**

494 **Answer: E.** The typical negative symptoms of schizophrenia are abulia, alogia, apathy, avolition and affective blunting. All the delusions, hallucinations and thought disorder symptoms are considered to be the positive symptoms of schizophrenia. **[D. pp. 166–7, 315–16]**

495 **Answer: D.** Some of the most important associations for these researchers are as follows:

- Brown and Harris – vulnerability factors for depression in women following life events.
- Brown and Birley – life events and schizophrenia.
- Holmes and Rahe – Holmes and Rahe Social Readjustment Rating Scale.
- Vaughan and Leff – expressed emotion and schizophrenic relapse.
- Wing and Brown – the Three Mental Hospitals Study.

[R. pp. 138–9, 375; M. p. 603]

496 **Answer: D.** Preoccupied attachment has been linked to insecure-ambivalent attachment in childhood. Adults displaying autonomous attachment are self-reliant, coherent in describing early experiences, objective and not defensive. It has been linked with secure attachment in childhood. Adults with a dismissing pattern of attachment appear to have few emotional memories of childhood. They tend to idealise caregivers and minimise the effects of traumatic events. This is thought to correspond to an insecure-avoidant attachment pattern in childhood. Adults with a pattern of unresolved attachment display gaps in their account of their childhood, particularly around traumatic events. This has been linked with disorganised childhood attachment. **[S. p. 67]**

497 Which one of the following psychiatric illnesses is more commonly diagnosed in people of higher social classes?

A. Alcohol dependence.

B. Bipolar disorder.

C. Depression.

D. Illicit drug use.

E. Schizophrenia.

498 In a 30-year-old man with a history of bipolar mood disorder presenting with severe flight of ideas, which of the following is less likely to be elicited in the mental state?

A. Alliteration.

B. Assonance.

C. Clang associations.

D. Derailment.

E. Punning.

499 A patient diagnosed with alcohol dependence syndrome has a long history of memory blackouts. He has developed memory loss for the events that happened during the alcohol binge drinking. In psychopathology terms, which of the following memory process is disturbed here?

A. Recall.

B. Recognition.

C. Registration.

D. Retention.

E. Retrieval.

500 The risk of developing obsessive compulsive disorder (OCD) has been found to be partly hereditary and is associated with Gilles de la Tourette syndrome (GDLT). Which one of the following statements concerning OCD is false?

A. Female relatives of GDLT probands are at higher risk of developing OCD.

B. Male relatives of GDLT probands are at higher risk of developing tics.

C. PET scans reveal decreased perfusion of the anterior cingulate.

D. The lifetime prevalence is 1.9–3%.

E. The gender ratio is equal.

497 **Answer: B.** Bipolar and eating disorders are more common in people from higher social classes. Psychopathy, alcohol dependence, illicit drug abuse, depression and schizophrenia are all more common in people from lower social classes. **[G. p. 61]**

498 **Answer: D.** In flight of ideas, the connections between various thoughts appear to be random. However, patients tend to make verbal associations of all kinds such as those listed in items A, B, C and E as well as rhyming, proverbs and clichés. Derailment is a formal thought disorder characteristic of schizophrenia. **[E. p. 1348; A. p. 251]**

499 **Answer: C.** Registration is an adequate perception of, comprehension of, and response to, events: it is an essential first step for proper memory formation. Alcohol-related amnesia and anterograde amnesia following head injury are two of the common clinical examples of impaired registration. **[D. pp. 50–1]**

500 **Answer: C.** The PET scans reveal increased perfusion of the anterior cingulate, basal ganglia, orbital and prefrontal cortex. **[R. p. 414]**

References

Note: References in the answer sections are given in the format: **[R. p. 156]**. This indicates that the topic relating to that particular MCQ may be found on page 156 of the text listed at 'R' below.

A. Johnstone EC, Freeman CPL, Zealley AK, editors. *Companion to Psychiatric Studies*. 6th ed. London: Churchill Livingstone; 1998.

B. Stein G, Wilkinson G, editors. *Seminars in General Adult Psychiatry*. London: Gaskell; 1998.

C. Eysenck M. *Simply Psychology*. Hove: Psychology Press; 1996.

D. Sims A. *Symptoms in the Mind: an introduction to descriptive psychopathology*. 2nd ed. London: WB Saunders Company Ltd; 1995.

E. Sadock BJ, Sadock VA, editors. *Kaplan & Sadock's Comprehensive Textbook of Psychiatry*. 7th ed. Philadelphia (PA): Lippincott, Williams & Wilkins; 2000.

F. Malhi, GS, Mitchell AJ. *Examination Notes in Psychiatry, Basic Sciences: a postgraduate text*. Oxford: Butterworth-Heinemann; 1999.

G. Puri BK, Hall AD. *Revision Notes in Psychiatry*. London: Arnold; 1998.

H. Buckley P, Bird J, Harrison G. *Examination Notes in Psychiatry: a postgraduate text*. 3rd ed. Oxford: Butterworth-Heinemann; 1995.

I. World Health Organization. *The ICD-10 Classification of Mental and Behavioural Disorders: clinical descriptions and diagnostic guidelines*. Geneva: World Health Organization; 1992.

J. American Psychiatric Association. *Diagnostic and Statistical Manual of Mental Disorders Fourth Edition: DSM-IV*. Washington (DC): American Psychiatric Association; 1994.

K. Kaplan HI, Sadock BJ, editors. *Comprehensive Textbook of Psychiatry*. 6th ed. Baltimore (MD): Williams & Wilkins; 1995.

L. Lishman WA. *Organic Psychiatry*. 3rd ed. Oxford: Blackwell Science; 1998.

M. Gelder MG, López-Ibor JJ, Andreasen N, editors. *New Oxford Textbook of Psychiatry*. Oxford: Oxford University Press; 2000.

N. Buckley P, Prewette D, Bird J, Harrison G, editors. *Examination Notes in Psychiatry*. 4th ed. London: Hodder Arnold; 2005.

O. Gross R. *Psychology: the science of mind and behaviour*. 4th ed. London: Hodder and Stoughton; 2001.

P. Sadock BJ, Sadock VA, editors. *Kaplan & Sadock's Comprehensive Textbook of Psychiatry*. 8th ed. Philadelphia (PA): Lippincott, Williams & Wilkins; 2005.

Q. Royal Pharmaceutical Society of Great Britain. *British National Formulary*. 53rd ed. London: Pharmaceutical Press; 2007.

R. Puri BK, Hall AD. *Revision Notes in Psychiatry*. 2nd ed. London: Arnold; 2004.

S. Wright P, Stern J, Phelan M. *Core Psychiatry*. London: WB Saunders; 2000.

T. Wright P, Stern J, Phelan M. *Core Psychiatry*. 2nd ed. Oxford: Elsevier Health Sciences; 2004.

U. Stahl SM. *Psychopharmacology of Antidepressants*. London: Martin Dunitz; 1997.

V. Taylor D, Paton C, Kerwin R. *The Maudsley Prescribing Guidelines*. 9th ed. London: Informa Health Care; 2007.

W. Bloch S. *An Introduction to the Psychotherapies*. 3rd ed. Oxford: Oxford University Press; 2006.

X. Bazire S. *Psychotropic Drug Directory 2005*. Salisbury: Fivepin Ltd; 2005.

Y. Fitzgerald MJT. *Neuroanatomy: basic and clinical*. 2nd ed. London: Balliere Tindall; 1992.

Z. Stahl SM. *Psychopharmacology of Antipsychotics*. London: Martin Dunitz; 1999.

AA. King DJ. *Seminars in Clinical Psychopharmacology*. London: Gaskell; 1995.

AB. Semple D, Smyth R, Burns J, Darjee R, McIntosh A. *Oxford Handbook of Psychiatry*. Oxford: Oxford University Press; 2005.

AC. Bruno FJ. *Psychology: a self-teaching guide*. New Jersey: John Wiley & Sons; 2002.

AD. Sadock BJ, Sadock VA, editors. *Kaplan and Sadock's Synopsis of Psychiatry: behavioral sciences/clinical psychiatry*. 9th ed. Philadelphia (PA): Lippincott, Williams & Wilkins; 2002.

AE. Munafo M. *Psychology for the MRCPsych*. 2nd ed. London: Arnold; 2002.

AF. Lawlor BA, editor. *Revision Psychiatry*. Dublin: MedMedia Ltd; 2001.

AG. Gelder MG, Gath D, Mayou R, Cowen P, editors. *Oxford Textbook of Psychiatry*. 3rd ed. Oxford: Oxford University Press; 1996.

AH. American Psychiatric Association. *Desk Reference to the Diagnostic Criteria from DSM-IV-TR*. Washington (DC): American Psychiatric Association; 2000.

AI. Bazire S. *Psychotropic Drug Directory 2001/2002*. Salisbury: Quay Books; 2001.

AJ. Mills, S. *Clinical Practice and the Law*. Dublin: Tottel; 2002.

AK. Kumar P, Clark M. *Clinical Medicine*. London: Balliere Tindall; 1994.

AL. Bannister R. *Brain's Clinical Neurology*. Oxford: Oxford University Press; 1985.

AM. Bloch S, Chodoff P, Green SA, editors. *Psychiatric Ethics*. 3rd ed. Oxford: Oxford University Press; 1999.

AN. Kuhse H, Singer P, editors. *A Companion to Bioethics*. Oxford: Blackwell; 1998.

AO. Talley N, O'Connor S. *Clinical Examination*. 2nd ed. Oxford: Blackwell Scientific Publications; 1992.

AP. Tantam D, Birchood M. *Seminars in Psychology and the Social Sciences*. London: Gaskell; 1994.

AQ. Taylor D, Paton C, Kerwin R. *The Maudsley Prescribing Guidelines 2005–2006*. 8th ed. Oxford: Taylor & Francis Group; 2005.

AR. Stahl S. *Essential Psychopharmacology: neuroscientific basis and practical applications*. 2nd ed. Cambridge: Cambridge University Press; 2000.

AS. Puri BK, Tyrer PJ. *Sciences Basic to Psychiatry*. 2nd ed. Edinburgh: Churchill Livingstone; 1998.

AT. Arikha N. *Passions and Tempers: a history of the humours*. New York: Ecco/HarperCollins; 2007.

AU. Malhi GS, Matharu MS, Hale AS. *Neurology for Psychiatrists*. London: Martin Dunitz Ltd; 2000.

AV. Kaplan HI, Sadock BJ, editors. *Synopsis of Psychiatry: behavioral sciences, clinical psychiatry*. 8th ed. Philadelphia (PA): Lippincott, Williams & Wilkins; 1998.

Index

(Q) refers to 'questions'; (A) to 'answers', key concepts or definitions.